DATE DUE

OCT 1 2 1993			
GAYLORD			PRINTED IN U.S.A.

ADVANCES IN HEALTH EDUCATION

Current Research
Volume 2

Edited by

Robert H. L. Feldman
and
James H. Humphrey

AMS PRESS, INC.
New York

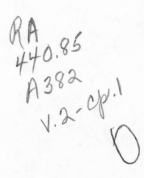

ADVANCES IN HEALTH EDUCATION *Current Research*

Copyright © 1989 by AMS Press, Inc.
All rights reserved

ISSN 0890-4073

Series ISBN: 0-404-63550-4
Vol. 2 ISBN: 0-404-63552-0
Library of Congress Catalog Card Number: 86-47857

Manufactured in the United States of America

AMS Press, Inc.
56 East 13th Street
New York, N.Y. 10003

All AMS books are printed on acid-free paper that meets the
guidelines for performance and durability of the Committee on
Production Guidelines for Book Longevity of the Council on
Library Resources.

CONTENTS

PREFACE

The second volume of *Advances in Health Education* presents a selection of current research in health education and state-of-the-art research reviews. The field of health education continues to exhibit multidisciplinary trends. Thus, the present volume reflects the great diversity within the field of health education.

The second volume examines such topics as patient education and the emerging area of gerontological health education. Smokeless tobacco, dental health, stress, and safety education are also included. In addition, the second volume contains selections on personal health, attitudes toward cancer, and the history of health education textbooks. Since worksite health is one of the fastest growing areas in health education we have included four reports on worksite health promotion and occupational health and safety.

In conjunction with AMS Press we intend to provide health education students and researchers with an annual series reporting original research investigating factors concerned with human health and health education. The volumes are intended to supplement and support journals reporting on similar topics. Papers eligible for inclusion in this and subsequent volumes must be (a) previously unpublished original research studies investigating selected aspects of health education. (b) state-of-the-art research reviews on topics of current interest with a substantial research literature base, or (c) theoretical papers presenting well-formulated but as yet untested models.

A volume of this nature would not be possible without the cooperation of many individuals. In this regard we wish to thank the contributors for presenting their work. In addition, we express our gratitude to the distinguished board of reviewers for giving their valuable time and excellent talents to this endeavor.

ABOUT THE EDITORS

Robert H. L. Feldman is Associate Professor and Director of the Program in Health Behavior, Department of Health Education, University of Maryland, College Park. Previously, he was on the faculty of Johns Hopkins University, School of Hygiene and Public Health. Dr. Feldman has published extensively in the areas of health behavior, health psychology, and worksite health (including co-authorship of *Occupational Health Promotion: Health Behavior in the Workplace*).

James H. Humphrey, Professor Emeritus at the University of Maryland, is the author of over 40 books and 200 articles and research reports. Ten of his books have been concerned with the areas of health and health education. A notable researcher, he was a charter member and first chairman-elect of the Research Council of the American School Health Association.

CONTRIBUTORS

Kenneth H. Beck, Department of Health Education, University of Maryland, College Park, Maryland

Randall R. Cottrell, Health and Nutrition Sciences, University of Cincinnati, Cincinnati, Ohio

Lorraine G. Davis, Department of School and Community Health, University of Oregon, Eugene, Oregon

George S. Everly, Harvard University, Cambridge, Massachusetts

Robert H. L. Feldman, Department of Health Education, University of Maryland, College Park, Maryland

Suzanne Laidlaw Feldman, Columbia, Maryland

Janet Fraser Hale, School of Nursing, Marymount University, Arlington, Virginia

Jerrold S. Greenberg, Department of Health Education, University of Maryland, College Park, Maryland

Jane M. Gutting, Educational Services, District 105, Yakima, Washington

Mary B. Harris, Department of Educational Foundations, University of New Mexico, Albuquerque, New Mexico

Roberta B. Hollander, Department of Physical Education and Recreation, Howard University, Washington DC

Joseph J. Lengermann, Department of Sociology, University of Maryland, College Park, Marykand

Massoumeh Majd-Jabbari, Indiana University, Bloomington, Indiana

Richard K. Means, Professor and Director of Health Education, Auburn University, Auburn, Alabama

R. Scott Olds, School of Health, Physical Education, and Recreation, Ithaca College, Ithaca, New York

John C. Ory, Division of Measurement and Research, University of Illinois, Urbana, Illinois

Jane A. Rankin, Department of Educational Foundations, University of New Mexico, Albuquerque, New Mexico

Martin Sherman, Loyola College in Maryland, Baltimore, Maryland

Kenneth J. Smith, University of Baltimore, Baltimore, Maryland

Donald B. Stone, Department of Health and Safety Studies, University of Illinois, Champaign, Illinois

Mohammad R. Torabi, Department of Applied Health Science, Indiana University, Bloomington, Indiana

Robert F. Valois, College of Education, University of Texas, Austin, Texas

C. Harold Veenker, Professor Emeritus of Health Education, Purdue University, West Lafayette, Indiana

BOARD OF REVIEWERS

1

ETHNIC, ACADEMIC, URBAN, AND RURAL SMOKELESS TOBACCO USE IN THE NORTHEASTERN UNITED STATES

R. Scott Olds

The purpose of this study is to measure ethnic, academic, urban, and rural prevalence of smokeless tobacco use by high school seniors in the State of New York. An anonymous and confidential questionnaire was administered to a 10% sample of each randomly selected secondary school in the State of New York. The questionnaire dichotomized smokeless tobacco into chewing tobacco and snuff so that more accurate representation of use could be presented. A total of 1,830 subjects successfully completed the questionnaire. Results indicate that Whites and Native Americans most frequently use smokeless tobacco. Further, subjects from rural settings more often are users of smokeless tobacco than urban subjects. Subjects with grade point averages of B and C more often are users of smokeless tobacco. The implications of this study suggest health education programs should be directed at these apparently high-risk groups. Further research is recommended to help delineate the use of smokeless tobacco in this country; the study protocol used in this study is recommended for future smokeless tobacco research efforts.

The apparent increase in smokeless tobacco use has raised concern among health professionals (United States Department of Health and Human Services, 1986). Smokeless tobacco use represents a significant health risk. It is not a safe alternative to smoking cigarettes; it can cause cancer and a number of noncancerous oral conditions, and can lead to nicotine addiction and dependence (USDHHS, 1986, p. vii).

Smokeless tobacco is available in several forms. The largest share of the market includes looseleaf chewing tobacco and moist snuff. Chewing tobacco is made from fire-cured tobacco leaves sweetened with sugars or licorice, and it is packaged in foil pouches ranging in size from 3.5 ounces to 11 ounces (Davis, 1986). The user of chewing tobacco places a "wad" or "quid" between the gum and jaw, usually toward the back of the oral cavity. The user is more likely to massage and manipulate the tobacco while sucking the tobacco juice and then expectorating than to actually chew it like bubble gum.

The second primary form of smokeless tobacco is moist snuff. Fine grain particles of tobacco, which can be enhanced with a myriad of flavorings and have a variety of nicotine potencies, are sold in 2.5-ounce tins. For instance, Skoal Bandits, which enjoys a large portion of the market, is sold in small teabag-like pouches to assist the beginner while offering a low dose of nicotine. The low dosage of nicotine may make the smokeless tobacco more palatable to the beginner with the intent to encourage their later use of stronger forms such as Copenhagen or Kodiak (David Brown Promotion Limited, 1985). The user of moist snuff places a "pinch" of tobacco in the gingival buccal area, between the cheek or lips and gum, and typically massages the tobacco between one-half hour to one hour (Olds, 1987). Between the two forms of smokeless tobacco just described, snuff often has the greater amount of nicotine and carcinogenic nitrosamines NNN and NNK (USDHHS, 1986).

In an attempt to identify the scope of smokeless tobacco use, the research completed to date often lacks random selection of subjects and is therefore subject to limited generalizability. The Surgeon General's Report on the Health Consequences of Using Smokeless Tobacco (USDHHS, 1986) recommended that further research utilizing adequate sample size was necessary to permit stratification by relevant variables including ethnicity, academic status, and urban and rural settings (p. 25). Further, the majority of research on smokeless tobacco has been completed in the Southeast, Southwest, and Midwest United States. The National Institutes of Health Consensus Development Conference on the Health Implications of Smokeless Tobacco Use (1986) stated: "Regional data on trends in the use of smokeless tobacco are not currently available."

Glover and Edwards (1985); Glover (1986); Marty, McDermott, and Williams (1986) and Bonaguro, Pugh, and Bonaguro (1986) found prevalence rates of smokeless tobacco use ranging from 11% to 33% for adolescent males. However, these studies did not report ethnic differences in use of smokeless tobacco and most often studied rural subjects.

Poulson, Lindenmuth, and Greer (1984), however, reported relatively high prevalence rates of smokeless tobacco use among urban adolescents in Colorado. Further, not a single study from the literature could be identified that presented data on the academic status of smokeless tobacco users. A paucity of data is available regarding the ethnic, academic, urban, and rural breakdown of smokeless tobacco use. Therefore, this study more clearly defines the scope of smokeless tobacco use and may assist the development of effective intervention techniques to decrease the incidence and prevalence of smokeless tobacco use in this age group, thus reducing the subsequent impact of this negative health behavior.

METHODOLOGY

A random selection of 10% of the secondary schools in the State of New York was drawn in order to achieve a representative sample of schools throughout the state. The 10% figure was selected because it was believed to provide a large enough pool of schools to more than adequately satisfy a study of this scope. As a result, 135 schools were contacted by mail and phone call correspondence. Results indicated that 96 schools, which represented 7.1% of the secondary schools in the state, agreed to participate.

The protocol for this study identified subjects in participating schools by classroom rather than by students. This technique had been used in previous research (McCarty & Krakow, 1985). Selection of subjects by classroom was a practical constraint of the design as the investigator believed that administrative and teacher support was more likely if intact classrooms were selected rather than individual students. Homerooms were preferred for data collection since less interruption of "in-class time" was required. However, flexibility of classroom designation was critical in gaining the principal's cooperation in administering the questionnaires.

Therefore, a 10% purposive sample by classroom in each participating school was drawn in order to strive for a representative sample (Rubinson & Neuten, 1987). This figure was selected to remain consistent across all participating schools and to provide a proportional number of subjects from each school's senior class.

Subjects were asked to voluntarily and anonymously provide their responses to the smokeless tobacco questionnaire. All subjects' responses were held in strict confidence by the researcher. Classroom teachers assisted with data collection and read an informed consent form to the subjects. Participation in the study presented no physical, emotional, psychological, or social risk to the subjects. Subjects could decline to participate at any time during completion of the questionnaire. The average completion time for the questionnaire was 20 minutes. Using Cronbach's alpha, the questionnaire had a high reliability coefficient of 0.83. A total of 1,895 questionnaires were administered and 1,830 subjects successfully completed the questionnaire for a return rate of 96.5%.

It is important to note that the questionnaire was designed to measure the primary forms of smokeless tobacco: chewing tobacco and snuff. This is believed to be an important aspect of this study because much of the previous research in this area does not delineate between these two primary forms of smokeless tobacco. Further, this delineation was recommended by the Surgeon General so that more accurate investigation of smokeless tobacco use could be undertaken (USDHSS, 1986). In this study, current smokeless tobacco users were defined as those who consumed smokeless tobacco two to three times a week (or more) in the last week.

This study served three purposes: (a) to identify if smokeless tobacco is related to various ethnic groups, (b) to identify if smokeless tobacco use was related to various levels of academic status, and (c) to determine if smokeless tobacco use was more prevalent in urban or rural settings. Therefore, the following hypotheses were formulated and stated in the null form:

1. No significant relationship exists between ethnic groups' prevalence of smokeless tobacco use.

2. No significant relationship exists between academic status and prevalence of smokeless tobacco use.

3. No significant difference exists between urban and rural prevalence of smokeless tobacco use.

Data analysis included descriptive presentation of data and the chi-square test of association (SPSSx Introductory Statistics Guide, 1986). For this study, smokeless tobacco use was considered a dichotomous variable. Analysis examined the prevalence of use between ethnic groups, varying levels of academic status, and urban and rural settings.

The level of statistical significance was set a priori at .05 (Hopkins & Glass, 1978). Findings that were statistically significant were further analyzed for practical significance by the phi-coefficient for 2 × 2 contingency tables and Cramer's V for tables larger than 2 × 2 (Torabi, 1986). Torabi (1986) stated that practical significance testing was important in applied disciplines such as health education. Practical significance testing would assist the provision of clues as to the proportion of variance in smokeless tobacco use being accounted for in this study by ethnicity, academic status, and urban and rural settings.

Data on prevalence of smokeless tobacco use is presented in several forms: smokeless tobacco (a composite of chewing tobacco use or snuff use), chewing tobacco use only, snuff use only, and concurrent use of both chewing tobacco and snuff. The smokeless tobacco variable has been created to provide a reflection of overall use of the two primary forms of smokeless tobacco—chewing tobacco or snuff. It is important the reader not be mislead to conclude that the smokeless tobacco variable over inflated the N because it has been created to avoid such a pitfall. Since chi-square does not allow for repeated frequencies for the smokeless tobacco variable, a computer program was written so that the smokeless tobacco category included subjects that were current users of chewing tobacco or snuff, thereby avoiding counting users more than once. The reader should keep this information in mind when reading tables that include the variable smokeless tobacco.

RESULTS

The sample was comprised of 55.4% males and 44.6% females. Subjects were predominantly White followed by Blacks, Hispanics, Asians, and Native Americans (See Figure 1). Figure 1 also presents a comparison of the ethnic breakdown of this sample as compared with state figures.

Findings indicated the majority of subjects reported grade point averages at the B+ (25.2%) and B (35.8%) level (See Figure 2). To increase the efficacy of data analysis, grade point averages were collapsed into a four point scale where 4 represented a grade of A. The mean grade point average was 2.9.

Results of the geographic spread of the sample revealed the distribution closely matched that described by the New York State Department of

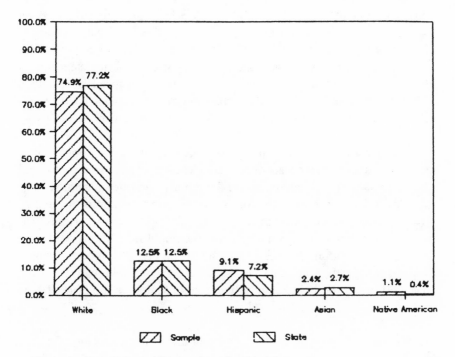

Figure 1   Description of Respondents by Ethnicity

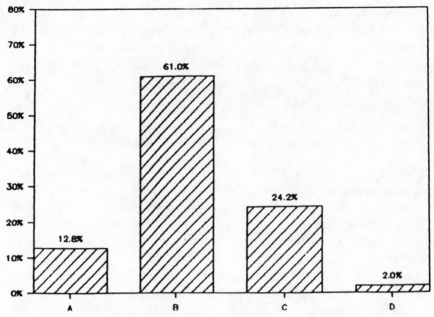

Figure 2. Respondents by Grade Point Average

Education's Booklet on Public and Nonpublic School Enrollment for 1985–86 (New York State Education Department, 1986). Further, the State Department of Education divides the state into 14 distinct regions. All regions were represented in the study. For analysis purposes, the four categories of hometown size, as indicated in Figure 3, were collapsed to create a dichotomous variable that included urban and rural categories. Figure 3 also provides a comparison of the sample by hometown size compared with state data.

To further verify that the sample was representative of the population of high school seniors in the State of New York, chi-square tests were performed to note any significant differences on the ethnicity and urban/rural settings variables. No proportionate differences were found for any of the ethnic groups except Native Americans. The sample of Native Americans was proportionally higher in this study than in the population. No proportionate differences were found between urban and rural breakdown of the sample as compared with state data. In summary, the sample had favorable characteristics of the population of high school seniors in the State of New York.

Prevalence of Use by Ethnicity. A statistically significant relationship was found between ethnicity and smokeless tobacco use (chi-square 15.1, *df* = 4,

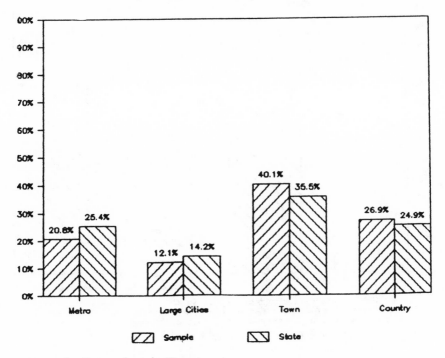

Figure 3.   Respondents by Hometown

$p = .004$) (See Figure 4), chewing tobacco (chi-square 14.45, $df = 4, p = .033$), and snuff use (chi-square 13.6, $df = 4, p = .008$) (See Figure 5); therefore, the hypothesis was rejected. Analysis of these statistically significant findings in prevalence of use by ethnic background was conducted to determine practical significance. Cramer's V indicated that 9% of the variation in use could be accounted for by this relationship for the smokeless tobacco group, 7.5% of the variation in chewing tobacco use, and 8.6% of the variation in snuff use. Native Americans and Whites represented the majority of users of smokeless tobacco, chewing tobacco, and snuff. Blacks and Hispanics did not indicate significant prevalence of use relative to the other ethnic groups. Asian subjects reported no use of either form of smokeless tobacco. Finally, examination of users of both chewing tobacco and snuff revealed no relationship between use and ethnicity (chi-square 8.7, $df = 4, p = .067$) (See Figure 5).

Prevalence of Use by Academic Status.   A statistically significant relationship was found between academic status and prevalence of smokeless tobacco use (chi-square 14.85, $df = 4, p = .005$) (See Figure 6), chewing tobacco use (chi-square 13.5, $df = 4$, snuff use (chi-square 12.84, $df = 4, p = .03$) and

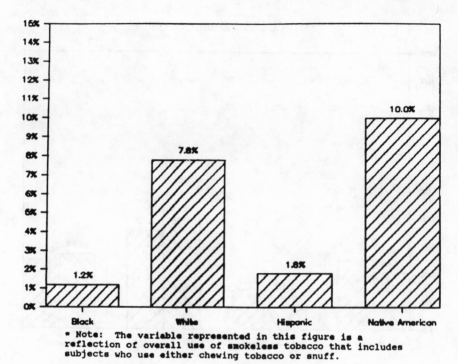

* Note: The variable represented in this figure is a reflection of overall use of smokeless tobacco that includes subjects who use either chewing tobacco or snuff.

Figure 4.   Smokeless Tobacco Use by Ethnicity

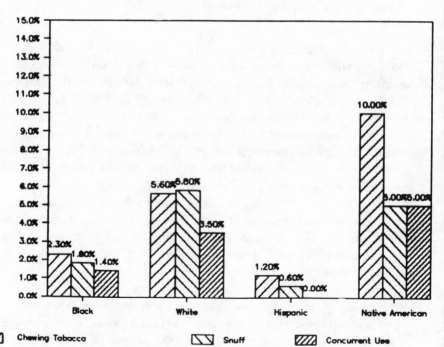

Figure 5.   Chewing Tobacco, Snuff, Concurrent Use

8

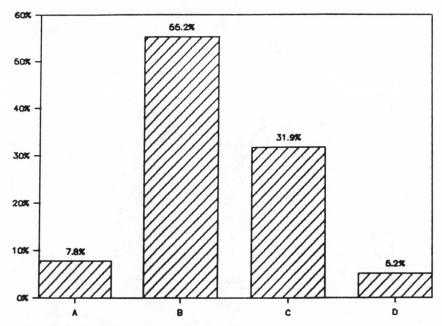

Figure 6. Smokeless Tobacco Use by GPA

concurrent use of chewing tobacco and snuff (chi-square 12.64, $df = 4, p = .01$) (See Figure 7); therefore, the hypothesis was rejected. The practical significance of this finding reveals that academic status accounted for 9% of the variation in this relationship as measured by Cramer's V for smokeless tobacco, 8.7% for chewing tobacco, 8.5% for snuff and 8.4% for use of both chewing tobacco and snuff. Subjects with grade point averages of B and C were more likely to be users of smokeless tobacco, chewing tobacco, snuff, and concurrent use of chewing tobacco and snuff.

Prevalence of Use by Urban and Rural Status. A statistically significant difference between urban and rural prevalence of smokeless tobacco use was found (chi-square 5.06, $df = 1, p = .02$) (See Figure 8), chewing tobacco use (chi-square 3.78, $df = 1, p = .05$) and snuff use (chi-square 4.05, $df = 1, p = .04$) (See Figure 9); therefore, the hypothesis was rejected. The practical significance of this finding reveals that hometown setting accounts for 5% of the variation in prevalence of smokeless tobacco use, 4.8% for chewing tobacco use and 5% for snuff use. No significant difference was found between urban and rural subjects' prevalence of concurrent use (chi-square 2.85, $df = 1, p = .09$). Rural subjects are more likely to be users of smokeless tobacco, chewing tobacco, and snuff than urban subjects (See Figure 9).

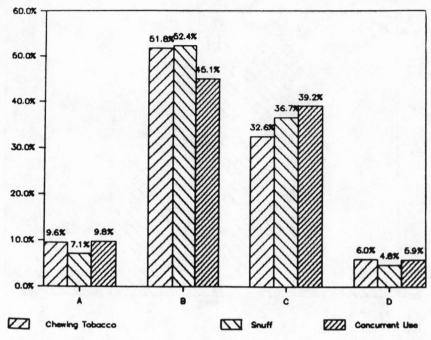

Figure 7. Chewing Tobacco, Snuff, Concurrent Use

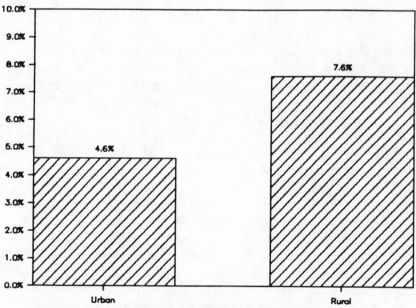

* Note: The variable represented in this figure is a reflection of overall use of smokeless tobacco that includes subjects who use either chewing tobacco or snuff.

Figure 8. Smokeless Tobacco Urban and Rural Uses

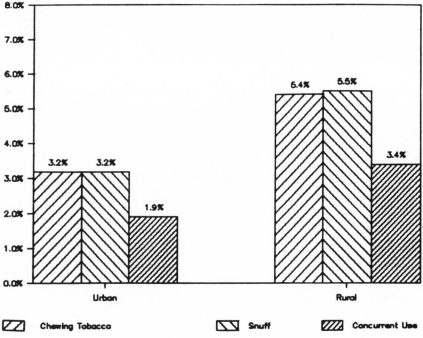

Figure 9.   Chewing Tobacco, Snuff, Concurrent Uses

DISCUSSION

The 1986 Surgeon General's Report on the Health Consequences of Using Smokeless Tobacco (USDHHS, 1986) indicated that the use of smokeless tobacco was apparently a habit predominantly of Whites. This study supports this finding, yet raises another question concerning the use of smokeless tobacco by Native Americans. It appears that further research is necessary to monitor prevalence of smokeless tobacco use with this subpopulation. The implications to health are significant given that Native Americans' use of alcohol (as a group) has been excessive and that the synergistic effects between alcohol and tobacco can be carcinogenic. This question is also important in terms of planning health education programs for this subpopulation as well as for the general population.

Inasmuch as data were collected via self-report, it is not surprising the mean grade point average was elevated. However, this is the first study to identify any relationship between academic status and smokeless tobacco use. Further study should be conducted in this area with an attempt to verify academic status.

The use of self-report admittedly has it limitations, but is also an efficient and practical data collection measure in health education. When resources are available, including financial and personnel support, consideration of chemical assays to measure nicotine levels as a by-product of smokeless tobacco use should be considered as a validity check with self-reported data collection in smokeless tobacco research. Further, examination of the bogus pipeline as an alternative should be considered as a validity check with self-reported data collection in smokeless tobacco research.

This study supports that of Glover and Edwards (1985), Marty, McDermott, and Williams (1986), and Bonaguro, Pugh, and Bonaguro (1986) that smokeless tobacco is a habit practiced primarily in rural settings. It seems important to consider focusing health education efforts in this area; however, it may be equally important not to ignore urban subjects lest we allow the smokeless tobacco habit to gain a strong foothold there, too.

In summary, further research is needed to determine how to effectively integrate education on smokeless tobacco into the school health curriculum, and educational programs in the community setting outside the traditional classroom. It is important that health educators respond to this health concern in a proactive manner, rather than a traditional reactive posture, which often seems to be a more difficult position to address. As Marty, McDermott, Young, and Guyton (1986) stated: "Health Education is presented with an opportunity they seldom get—that of altering the course of a negative health behavior that is still within the realm of prevention control" (p. 31). In conclusion, the following anonymous quote accurately reflects the position health educators should encourage all people to take with smokeless tobacco: "Some things are better eschewed than chewed, and tobacco is one of them."

REFERENCES

Bonaguro, J. A., Pugh, M., & Bonaguro, E. W. (1986). Multivariate analysis of smokeless tobacco use by adolescents in grades four through twelve. *Health Education, 17*(2), 4–8.

Davis, E. (1986). Types of Smokeless Tobacco. National Institutes of Health Consensus Development Conference. Bethesda, Maryland.

David Brown Promotion Limited (1985). Introduction of Skoal Bandits, Cranleigh, Scotland: 1–4

Glover, E. D. (1986). *Prevalence of smokeless tobacco.* National Institutes of Health Consensus Development Conference. Bethesda, MD.

Glover, E. D., & Edwards, S. W. (1985). *Prevalence of smokeless tobacco use in Oklahoma public schools.* Unpublished manuscript, East Carolina University, Greenville, NC.

Hopkins, R. D., & Glass, G. V. (1978). *Basic statistics for the behavioral sciences.* Englewood Cliffs, NJ: Prentice-Hall.

Marty, P. J., McDermott, R. J., & Williams, R. (1986). Patterns of smokeless tobacco use in a population of high school students. *American Journal of Public Health, 76*(2), 190–192.

Marty, P. J., McDermott, R. J., Young, M., & Guyton, R. (1986). Prevalence and psychosocial correlates of dipping and chewing behavior in a group of rural high school students. *Health Education, 17*(2), 28–32.

McCarty, D., & Krakow, M. (1985, January). More than just a pinch: The use of smokeless tobacco among Massachusetts students. Report by the Massachusetts Department of Public Health, division of Drug Rehabilitation.

National Institutes of Health Consensus Development Conference on the Health Implications of Smokeless Tobacco Use. (1986). Consensus statement. USPHS.

New York State Education Department. (1986). *Racial/Ethnic Distribution of Public Schools Students.* Albany, NY.

New York State Education Department. (1986). *Public and Nonpublic School Enrollment.* Albany, NY.

Olds, R. S. (1987). *Patterns and prevalence of smokeless tobacco use by high school seniors in the state of New York.* Unpublished manuscript, Ithaca College, Ithaca, NY.

Poulson, T. C., Lindenmuth, J. E., & Greer, R. O. (1984). A comparison of the use of smokeless tobacco in rural and urban teenagers. *Ca-A Cancer Journal for Clinicians, 34*(5), 248–261.

SPSSx Introductory Statistics Guide, (1986). SPSS Inc., Chicago, IL.

Rubinson, L., & Neutens, J. J. (1987). Research Techniques for the Health Sciences. NY: MacMillan Publishing Company.

Torabi, M. R. (1986). How to estimate practical significance in health education research. *Journal of School Health, 56*(7), 232–233.

United States Department of Health and Human Services. (1986). *Surgeon General's Report on the Health Consequences of Using Smokeless Tobacco.* USPHS. Washington, DC: U.S. Government Printing Office.

2

CONSTRUCT VALIDATION OF A CANCER ATTITUDE SCALE BY MULTIVARIATE ANALYSES

Mohammad R. Torabi

Massoumeh Majd-Jabbari

C. Harold Veenker

The purpose of this study was to provide construct validity evidence for the "Three Component Cancer Attitude Scale for College Students" by examining underlying factor structure of the students' attitudes toward cancer and cancer prevention. The attitude scale was administered to a representative sample of over 1000 undergraduate college students in five major universities across the United States. The collected data were subjected to multivariate analyses including factor analysis (FA), and cluster analysis (CA). Results of FA and CA, which were consistent, identified five factors/clusters that describe the construct of students' attitudes toward prevention of cancer. The scale was found to be valid, and the findings supported the specificity principle in attitudinal measurement. This means that attitude items are more interrelated with respect to attitudinal object (content) than the component structure of attitudes.

Much of the attitude research in recent years has been directed at the attitude-behavior relationship. One school of thought believes that attitude and behavior are related causally in a sequential chain, that a reciprocal relationship exists (Bagozzi, 1978). Earlier theorists have suggested that attitudes and behavior are basically independent; that is, any kind of attitude could exist in conjunction with any kind of behavior, even toward the same object. Despite various claims, however, most studies have yielded inconclusive results. Consequently, many researchers now believe that this disagreement is due mainly to the absence of conceptual underpinnings for the attitude construct.

Attitude was commonly defined by some researchers as a learned predisposition to respond to an object in a consistently positive or negative way. In this view, attitude becomes a unidimensional concept that pertains only to the individual's feelings of like or dislike for a particular object. This single-component model recognizes attitude only as affect, ignoring other possible indicants of behavior. A problem then arises as to its ability to predict behavior from single attitude scores that place individuals at a particular point between two extremes.

More recent research has come to question this approach as over simplified unidimensionality. Rosenberg and Hovland (1960), Bagozzi (1978), Fishbein (1967), Kothandapani (1971b), Ostrom (1969), and Veenker and Torabi (1983) support a multidimensional approach that includes cognition (belief) and conation (intention to act), as well as affect (feeling), as components of attitude. The relationship of these components with each other and with actual behavior is of prime importance to the multidimensional approach of attitude; the affective component accounts for the degree of emotional attraction toward an attitudinal object; the cognitive component perceives the relationship between the attitudinal object and other objects; and cognition describes "belief about the object, characteristics of the object, and relationships of the objects with other objects" (Ostrom, 1969, p. 16).

Several studies have been conducted to provide empirical support for a multidimensional conceptualization of attitude. Ostrom (1969), for example, investigated the attitudes of 189 undergraduate students toward the Church, using cognitive, affective, and conative scales. Similarly, Kothandapani's study (1971a) measured attitudes toward birth control among 100 low-income married black women, some users and some nonusers of contraceptives. The results of both investigations revealed that the correlations obtained by the attitude component scores furnished evidence for the convergent and discriminant validity for all three components. However, a reanalysis of both sets of data show that only the Ostrom study distinctively supports a multicomponent attitude model. Bagozzi (1978) also concludes that the three components of attitude share a common variance and perhaps could be regarded as parts of a single underlying construct of attitude.

Health related behavior, like all other human behavior, is largely determined by attitudes. Individuals are likely to adopt those health behaviors and practices that they already favor. This has significant implications for public health education, one area of which is cancer prevention. A recent epidemiology study (American Cancer Society, 1983) has associated certain behavior directly with cancer deaths: smoking, poor nutrition, having multiple sexual partners and/or early sexual activity, and excessive alcohol use. How individuals feel about the prevention of cancer, what they believe about it, and the extent to which they intend to act upon those feelings and beliefs, all significantly affect their behavior in preventing cancer.

To measure cancer attitudes in their three components, separately and in total, a valid and reliable instrument was developed by Torabi (1985) and Torabi and Seffrin (1986). This Likert-type instrument was constructed according to a table of specifications identifying three conceptual areas: general information about cancer, cancer prevention, and cancer detection. The 30-item attitude scale consisting of three subscales with 10 conceptually comparable items in each of the subscales. Items 1 to 10, 11 to 20, and 21 to 30 measure the components of feeling, belief, and intention to act, respectively. (See Table 1) Evidence of validity was demonstrated through various statistical analyses of the data. The reliability coefficients of the total scale were .94 and .82, using Cronbach alpha and the split-half method, respectively. The subscales of feeling, belief, and intention to act also showed high reliabilities, ranging from .70 to .93. Beyond the above-mentioned data describing scale performance, this report presents the results of multivariate analyses as evidence of the construct validity of the instrument.

METHOD

The attitude scale was administered to 1040 undergraduate male and female students in five major universities in the U.S. Almost half the participants were 19 to 20 years old. Over 17% were 18 or younger, less than 9% were 23 years old and older, and the remainder were in the 21–22 year age group. About two-thirds of the students were equally divided among freshmen and sophomores; 21% were juniors, and the smallest number, 15%, were seniors. Approximately 78% of the students were from the Midwest, with the rest representing other parts of the U. S. and other countries. The subjects represented most university academic fields.

To reveal the underlying structure of attitudes toward cancer prevention, the data were subjected to two multivariate statistical techniques: factor analysis (FA), and cluster analysis (CA). The maximum likelihood method was employed in FA because of two certain advantages (SAS User's Guide, 1982). This method gives better and more distinct estimates than its more commonly used competitor, principal factor analysis, especially in large samples; and maximum likelihood allows testing the hypothesis about the number of common factors.

TABLE 1
Instruction, Items, and Scoring of a Cancer Attitude Scale

Please read each statement carefully. Record your immediate reaction to the statement by darkening the letter on the answer sheet which best describes how well you agree or disagree with the idea according to the following scale:

a = Strongly Agree (SA)
b = Agree (A)
c = Undecided (U)
d = Disagree (D)
e = Strongly Disagree (SD)

1. I would enjoy talking with a cancer patient.
2. I feel sorry for cancer patients.
3. I hate to smoke because of its cancer causing effects.
4. If one feels healthy, s/he does not need a physical checkup.
5. I enjoy smoking regardless of the consequences.
6. The idea of breast examination by a physician is embarrassing.
7. It is enjoyable having sexual intercourse with multiple partners.
8. Colorectal cancer is an embarrassing disease.
9. I feel sorry for those people who have skin cancer.
10. Young people do not have to be worried about prostate cancer.
11. Cancer is a mysterious disease.
12. Cancer is the worst disease known to mankind.
13. I think cancer is not a preventable disease.
14. Breast self-examination is a waste of time.
15. Because of the carcinogenic (cancer causing) effect of tobacco, its public use should be prohibited by law.
16. Breast cancer is exclusively a woman's problem.
17. I believe that uterine cancer is a rare type of cancer.
18. It is difficult for me to talk about colorectal cancer.
19. I believe that skin cancer is a deadly form of cancer.
20. The rectal exam is not an acceptable technique for checking the prostate gland.
21. I would rather not hear about cancer.
22. In order to avoid cancer, I would do almost anything to protect myself.
23. I prefer to work in a healthy environment, even if it means taking a lower salary.
24. I intend to see my physician anytime I observe any unusual changes or when suspicious symptoms appear.
25. I intend to stay away from smoking cigarettes for the rest of my life.
26. I intend to do breast self-examination once a month.
27. I would encourage my friends to have a regular pap test.
28. For purposes of preventing colorectal cancer, I intend to encourage my family to have a diet high in fiber.
29. I intend to do whatever I can to protect myself against skin cancer.
30. I intend to encourage my close friends to be concerned about their prostate gland.

Scoring: For items 2, 4, 14, 16 to 21, strongly agree equals 1 point, agree 2 points, undecided 3 points, disagree 4 points and strongly disagree 5 points; for the remaining items, reverse the order of values assigned to alternatives with strongly agree equalling 5 points and strongly disagree equalling 1 point. The higher score is interpreted as more positive attitudes toward cancer prevention. This scale is named Torabi-Seffrin Cancer Attitude Scale. For further information, contact the primary author.

To make a cluster analysis, the "VARCLUS" procedure was used (SAS User's Guide, 1982). This procedure is a reduction method that places a set of variables into disjoint (nonoverlapping) clusters in such a way that each cluster can be interpreted as essentially congruent. A component was computed for each cluster in an effort to maximize the sum across clusters of the variance of the original variables that is accounted for by the cluster components. As a variable-reduction method, VARCLUS is a type of oblique component analysis. The cluster structure is analogous to the factor structure, presenting the correlation between each variable and each cluster component. The intercluster correlations correspond to interfactor correlations; they are correlations among cluster components. The VARCLUS technique essentially permits a large set of variables to be replaced by a set of cluster components with little loss of information. In conducting cluster analysis, a tree diagram known as a dendogram or phenogram was obtained using the "TREE" procedure (SAS User's Guide, 1982). This procedure has the capability of identifying disjoint clusters at a specified level on the tree.

RESULTS

The initial factor solution identified five statistically significant factors (chi-square $= 753.669, p = <.01$). All but one factor had eigenvalues greater than one. Figure 1 describes the Scree plot of eigenvalues against the number of factors.

The plot shows a fairly constant slope subsequent to the first five factors, accounting for 88.45% of the total variance. This implies that the remaining factors extract either random errors or substantially meaningless factors. The item scores of the total scale were then subjected to varimax rotation for the extracted five factors. The resulting factor loadings of the thirty items are presented in Table 2.

Factor loadings of .40 or above were used as a minimum criterion in identifying the scale items associated with each of these five factors. The first factor, labelled "intention for prevention," is identified with items 5, 22, 28, 29, and 30 and accounts for 20.35% of the variance. These items deal with primary and secondary prevention of cancer. Factor 2, called "primary prevention," is explained by items 3, 5, 15, and 25. These items come from the subscales measuring all three components of attitude. This factor pertains specifically to attitudes toward cigarette smoking in relation to its cancer-causing effects, and accounts for 20.2% of the variance. Factor 3 explains 17.4% of the variance and is measured by items 4, 6, 8, 10, and 14. These items, representing the two subscales of feeling and belief, essentially

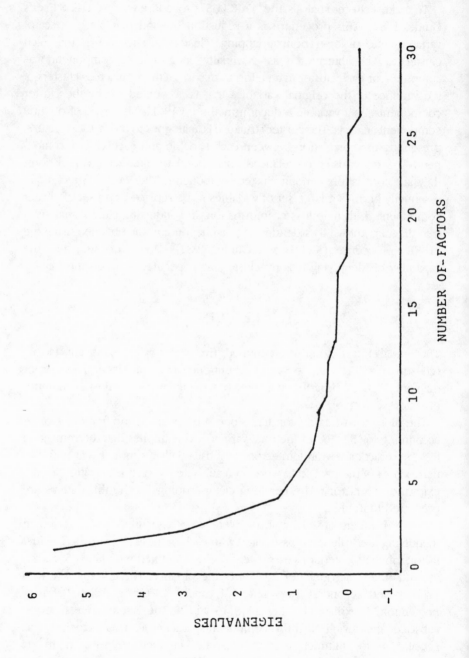

Figure 1.   Scree Plot of Eigenvalues

TABLE 2
Factor Pattern After Varimax Rotation

	Factor 1	Factor 2	Factor 3	Factor 4	Factor 5
1	.21	.11	.17	.25	.04
2	.02	−.09	.00	−.66	.91
3	−.17	.60	.04	.70	−.11
4	.16	.01	.40	.62	−.02
5	.49	.80	.05	−.06	.00
6	.11	−.09	.40	.02	.09
7	.01	.06	.22	.37	−.05
8	−.06	.02	.41	.18	.07
9	−.13	−.06	.03	.04	.63
10	.10	.03	.42	.02	.02
11	−.03	−.01	.17	.04	.27
12	−.09	−.04	.20	−.04	.35
13	.01	.05	.28	−.02	.06
14	.15	.01	.45	.23	−.03
15	.08	.40	−.08	.03	−.03
16	.00	.03	−.28	.07	.09
17	.01	.04	−.36	.18	−.02
18	.06	−.09	.34	−.17	−.01
19	.18	−.01	−.09	−.13	−.04
20	.02	.03	−.19	.02	−.04
21	.16	.05	.36	.13	.03
22	.55	.31	.03	.04	−.16
23	.32	.26	.08	.17	−.07
24	.39	.11	.22	.25	−.11
25	.16	.75	.09	.00	.04
26	.21	.03	.05	.76	.05
27	.34	−.05	.23	.59	−.03
28	.52	.11	.12	.30	−.05
29	.68	.13	.07	−.01	.00
30	.55	.07	.07	.24	−.06
Variance Explained by Each Factor					
Unweighted	2.02	1.99	1.74	1.57	1.53

express feelings of negativism toward and embarrassment by cancer, certain cancer detection techniques, and physical checkup. Because of this underlying content, this factor is labelled "negativism toward cancer." The fourth factor is associated with five items and explains 15.3% of the variance. Items 2–4, 26, and 27 pertain to early detection techniques and prevention. Factor 4 is thus identified as "general cancer prevention." The fifth factor also explains 15.2% of the variance. The content of two items linked to this factor,

2 and 9, embody sympathy toward people who are suffering from the disease. Consequently, factor 5 is named "sympathy for cancer patients."

The second multivariate analysis of attitudes toward cancer prevention involved cluster analysis. The VARCLUS procedure, a type of oblique component analysis, yielded five disjoint clusters summarized in Table 3.

Cluster 4 with 11 items and cluster 5 with only 3 items are the largest and smallest clusters, respectively. Cluster 1 contains 7 items; cluster 2, 4 items; and cluster 3, 5 items. The table also reveals that only about 37% of the variance is explained by these five clusters, or less than half the variance accounted for by the five factors generated through factor analysis (Table 4).

As was the case in factor analysis, only cluster components of .40 and above were considered for determining the cluster members. According to Table 4, cluster 1 unites items 1, 7, 24, 26, 27, 28, and 30. These 7 items, representing all three attitude components (feeling, belief, and intention to act), are linked to early detection techniques. In reference to its item content, the label "secondary prevention" is justified for this cluster. The second cluster consists of 4 items: 3, 5, 15, and 25. As with cluster 1, these items belong to all three attitude subscales. Cluster 2, being identical to factor 2, is called the cluster of "primary prevention." Cluster 3 unites items 2, 9, 11, and 12, which essentially measure sympathy toward cancer patients. This cluster derives items from the feeling and belief subscales only, and is parallel to factor 5. Items 4, 6, 8, 10, 14, 16, 17, and 21 are coalesced in the fourth cluster. Again, these items cut across all three components and express negative attitudes toward cancer. Consequently, the cluster "negativism toward cancer" is formed. This cluster is analogous to factor 3.

TABLE 3
Oblique Principal Component Cluster Analysis
Cluster Summary for 5 Clusters

Cluster	Member	Cluster Variation	Variation Explanation	Proportion Explained	Second Eigenvalue
1	7	7.00	2.70	.39	1.05
2	4	4.00	2.27	.57	.80
3	5	5.00	1.98	.39	1.04
4	11	11.00	2.41	.22	1.14
5	3	3.00	1.71	.57	.76

TOTAL VARIATION EXPLAINED = 11.0588
PROPORTION = 0.368627

TABLE 4
Oblique Principal Component Cluster Analysis
Cluster Structure

Cluster	1	2	3	4	5
1	.47	.14	−.01	.23	.22
2	−.08	−.13	.79	.05	−.12
3	.21	.76	−.16	.08	.31
4	.24	.06	.01	.50	.12
5	.11	.83	−.07	.07	.26
6	.15	−.06	.10	.50	.06
7	.41	.09	−.03	.27	.13
8	.18	.03	.11	.53	−.00
9	−.07	−.12	.73	.07	−.16
10	.15	.07	.03	.54	.10
11	.04	−.03	.59	.12	−.00
12	−.04	−.06	.65	.14	−.11
13	.06	.05	.15	.32	.05
14	.33	.06	−.004	.61	.18
15	.07	.56	−.08	−.03	.22
16	.10	.02	.12	.40	.04
17	−.19	.01	−.08	−.48	−.05
18	−.17	−.08	−.21	−.06	.07
19	−.01	.03	−.21	−.06	.07
20	−.02	.01	−.03	−.26	.04
21	.29	.08	.04	.49	.14
22	.34	.36	−.20	.01	.82
23	.33	.29	−.07	.12	.68
24	.59	.18	−.09	.10	.35
25	.18	.83	−.09	.10	.35
26	.72	.08	.03	.23	.21
27	.76	.04	−.04	.35	.26
28	.67	.18	−.05	.21	.44
29	.38	.22	−.06	.14	.76
30	.65	.16	−.09	.17	.38

The final cluster groups items 22, 23, 28, and 29. All of these items relate exclusively to the intention subscale and are comparable to the items constituting factor 1. Following the label given to this factor, cluster 5 becomes "intention for general cancer prevention."

The dendogram, produced from the TREE procedure, is presented in Figure 2.

At level 1 Figure 2 shows that all 30 items are assembled together, forming one cluster. At the next level, two nonoverlapping clusters are formed,

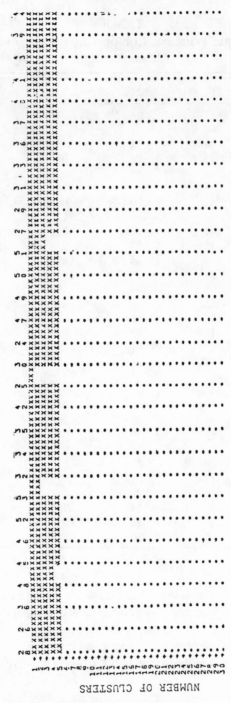

NUMBER OF CLUSTERS

Figure 2.   Oblique Principal Component Clustering

containing 13 and 17 items, respectively. At level 3, the cluster with 17 items remains unchanged. A further splitting occurs only in the 13-item cluster, dividing it into 2 clusters with 8 and 5 items each. At level 4, the first cluster is divided into two clusters, which, along with the remaining two clusters, form a four-cluster level. Finally, at the last level, five disjoint clusters, containing 5-item groups emerge.

DISCUSSION

While very similar groupings of items were produced independently by FA and CA, these item groups were not congruent with any one of the three components identified in attitude structure. In general, the items in each group function across all three components and do not reflect any specific subscale. This result is consistent with those of an earlier study, which found that "focus of attitudinal measures is not so much in a component of attitude as it is in the subsets of attitudinal objects within a conceptual area of health behavior." (Veenker & Torabi, 1983). Moreover, formation of five groups of items determined by FA and CA has significant implication. These item groups could be utilized for selected factor measurement in subsequent attitude studies.

It is clear that the instrument functions effectively to measure the affective, cognitive, and conative components of attitudes toward cancer and its prevention. The component structure obviously does not correspond to the structure unfolded by the multivariate item analyses. In fact, this disparity lends further support to the assertion that attitudinal items, rather than relating generally to the component structure of attitudes, intercorrelate instead in direct relation to attitudinal object. (Veenker & Torabi, 1983).

These results support the suggestion that the composition of the factor or cluster structure associated with college students' attitudes toward cancer and cancer prevention has potential value for educators and researchers concerned with cancer prevention.

REFERENCES

American Cancer Society (1983). *Cancer causes and prevention: clues from epidemiology* [Slide set for Professional Education]. A.C.S. Code #3809.

Bagozzi, R. P. (1978). The construct validity of the affective, behavioral and cognitive components of attitude by analysis of covariance structures. *Multivariate Behavioral Research, 13,* 9–31.

Fishbein, M. (1967). Attitudes and the prediction of behavior. In M. Fishbein (Ed.), *Readings in Attitude Theory and Measurement* (pp. 3–13). New York: John Wiley and Sons, Inc.

Harding, J., & Kuther, B. (1954). Prejudice and ethnic relations. *Handbook of Social Psychology* (p. 1023).

Kothandapani, V. (1971a). *A psychological approach to the prediction of contraceptive behavior* (pp. 1–93). Carolina Publication Center: University of North Carolina.

Kothandapani, V. (1971b). Validation of feeling, belief, and intention to act as three components of attitude and their contribution to prediction of contraceptive behavior. *Journal of Personality and Social Psychology, 19,* 321–333.

Ostrom, T. M. (1969). The relationship between the affective behavioral and cognitive components of attitude. *Journal of Experimental Social Psychology, 5*(1), 12–30.

Rosenberg, M. J., & Hovland, C. I. (1960). Cognitive, affective, and behavioral components of attitudes. In M. J. Rosenberg, et al. (Eds.), *Attitude Organization and Change.* New Haven, CT: Yale University Press.

Statistical Analysis System. (1982). *SAS User's Guide: Statistics* (pp. 313, 461–473, 450–460). Cary, North Carolina: Author.

Subkoviak, M. J. (1975). The use of multidimensional scaling in educational research. *Review of Educational Research, 45*(3), 387–423.

Torabi, M. R. (1985, October). *Cancer attitude scale.* Paper presented at America School Health Association, Little Rock, AR. (1986)

Torabi, M. R., & Seffrin, J. R. *Cancer Attitude Scale.* Journal of School Health.

Veenker, C. H., & Torabi, M. R. (1983). Multivariate Analysis of Dimensionality in Health Attitude Structure. *Health Education, 14*(7), 16–21.

3

A STUDY OF THE RELATIONSHIP BETWEEN COGNITIVE AND AFFECTIVE TAXONOMIC PERFORMANCE IN HEALTH EDUCATION

Robert F. Valois

John C. Ory

Donald B. Stone

To provide health educators with information regarding the relationship between cognitive and affective student performance, this study was conducted at a midwestern university.

Subjects for this study included approximately 90 students from two required personal health classes in the instrumentation phase. Subjects in the experimental phase consisted of approximately 506 students. The control group included 110 students from six mathematics and two English classes, while the experimental group consisted of 396 students from all required personal health classes. The *required* (for graduation) personal health course was taught by four instructors from the same department within the university. All four instructors utilized the same organizational structure in regard to course objectives, required texts, evaluation, and grading.

A 138-item Personal Health Knowledge and Attitude instrument was utilized to assess personal health knowledge and attitudes. The instrument was developed by using the hierarchical structure of the Taxonomy of Educational Objectives, Cognitive and Affective Domains, for the topics of alcohol use, smoking behavior, stress management, exercise-rest, and nutrition weight control. The instrument was evaluated by a panel of educational psychologists and a panel of health educators and was declared construct and content valid.

The research design for this study was a repeated measures, pretest, posttest experimental-control group design with subjects matched across time. Data analysis was divided into two phases. Phase I pertained to the evaluation of cognitive and affective outcomes of the required course in personal health. Statistical procedures for this phase utilized separate two-way ANOVAS (time × group) for cognitive, affective subscales, and also for total scores for these two scales. The second phase dealt with the relationship between the affective and cognitive taxonomic performance in personal health education. An analysis was performed in this phase on the affective subscale mean scores across four cognitive taxonomic levels, followed by four univariate F-tests using Wilks Lambda (U-Statistic) to determine significant mean differences.

Based on the results of this study a relationship does exist between the cognitive and affective taxonomies. They are parallel in nature, and there is an intimate relationship between cognitive learning and affective internalization. This relationship exists at the knowledge/receiving levels as well as the analysis-synthesis/organization levels.

By teaching to the higher levels of cognition a health educator may also be developing positive attitudes and vice versa. Health educators may wish to acknowledge these results since the goals of health education are to increase cognition, develop positive health attitudes and ultimately influence positive life-style behaviors.

The authors of the Taxonomy of Educational Objectives (Bloom, 1956; Krathwohl, 1964) refer to this theoretical concept as cognitive and affective domains. They provide a classification system for educational objectives based on components of each of these domains. This system can be viewed as a hierarchy of objectives: as an individual's thinking advances through a domain, the level of learning and/or internalization demonstrated increases in sophistication.

The cognitive domain relates to the individual's ability to deal with knowledge and factual information from an intellectual perspective. It is arranged into six major classes, which move from simple to complex. The classes are: knowledge, comprehension, application, analysis, synthesis, and evaluation.

The affective domain involves personal interests, attitudes, values, and the development of appreciations and adequate adjustments. Again a hierarchy exists ranging from the simple to the complex. The following is the classification of the affective domain: receiving, responding, valuing, organization, and value complex.

A close relationship exists between the cognitive and affective taxonomies; they are parallel in nature; and there is an intimate relationship between cognitive and affective learning. This relationship is operative at the knowledge-receiving levels as well as the analysis/synthesis-organization levels. As the author of the Affective Taxonomy (Krathwohl, 1964) points out:

The two domains are tightly intertwined. Each affective behavior has a cognitive behavior counterpart of some kind and vice versa. An objective in one domain has a counterpart in the opposite domain, though often we do not take cognizance of it. . . . Each domain is sometimes used as a means to the other, though the more common route is from the cognitive to the affective. Theory statements exist which permit us to express one in terms of the other and vice versa. (p. 62)

As the above quotation indicates, affective qualities may be assessed indirectly through the use of traditional cognitive techniques. What is not clear, however, is how the levels of the two domains related to one another. Is there a correspondence between "achievement" at different levels of the two domains? Do individuals achieving at the higher levels of one domain also achieve at the higher levels of the other?

Over the years, studies have been conducted wherein the researchers have attempted to validate the hierarchical structure of the cognitive and affective domains (Stroker & Kroop, 1964; Lewy, 1968). In general, the research has supported the hierarchy of levels within both taxonomies as they were originally hypothesized. What is conspicuously missing in the health education literature is research investigating the hierarchical relationship between performance in both domains of the Taxonomy of Educational Objectives.

PURPOSE

The purpose of this study was to examine the relationship between cognitive and affective taxonomic performance of undergraduate students in a required personal health course at a midwestern university. Personal Health 1200 has been a general education requirement for a substantial part of the university's history. Beginning the fall semester 1981, this basic health class became a graduation requirement. As a theoretical framework for conducting this investigation, the Cognitive and Affective Domains of the Taxonomy of Educational Objectives (Bloom, 1956; Krathwohl, 1964) were utilized. These two domains were chosen on the basis of their hierarchical structure and their parallel nature; and because they both have in their lower categories, simple concrete learning that serves as "building blocks" for more sophisticated learning.

A personal health course was chosen for the context of the study because of the goals and objectives of personal health education. The chief goals of health education are threefold according to Bedworth and Bedworth (1978):

(a) the acquisition of health knowledge, (b) the improvement or reinforcement of health attitudes, and (c) the improvement or reinforcement of health behavior. Changes in knowledge and attitudes are acknowledged as "precursors" to appropriate behavior.

METHODOLOGY

This study consisted of an instrumentation phase and an experimental phase. The instrumentation phase consisted of developing the personal health knowledge and attitude instrument, and pilot-testing it in two required personal health classes similar to the classes being used in the experimental phase. The experimental phase consisted of utilizing the Personal Health Knowledge and Attitude Questionnaire in assessing the effects of a basic personal health course on the cognition and affect of college students. The relationship between cognitive and affective outcomes of a required personal health course at the college level was also determined.

Instrumentation

The primary instrument employed in this study was an 80-item Personal Health Knowledge and Attitude Questionnaire developed by the investigator in the pilot phase. This instrument consisted of five sub-scale topics: Nutrition-Weight Control, Stress Management, Exercise-Rest, Alcohol Use, and Smoking Behavior. The knowledge section of the instrument contained 30 multiple choice items, each having four response alternatives, and 10 multiple true-false items each having five cognitive statements. This scale was developed from a table of specifications utilizing Bloom's Taxonomy of Educational Objectives, Cognitive Domain.

Descriptions (working definitions) of the major categories of the Cognitive and Affective Domains of the Taxonomy of Educational Objectives can be located in Figures 1 and 2 respectively. Knowledge items were selected to represent the knowledge, comprehension, application, and analysis-synthesis levels of the cognitive taxonomy for all five subscale topics. Each of the five subscales contained eight knowledge items, two items for each of the four levels of the cognitive taxonomy.

The attitude section of the instrument consisted of 40, five-point Likert Scale items. The five response choices to each attitudinal item included: strongly disagree, disagree, undecided, agree, and strongly agree, in that order. This scale was developed from a table of specifications utilizing Krathwohl's Taxonomy of Educational Objectives, Affective Domain. Attitude

Figure 1

Major Categories in the Cognitive Domain of the Taxonomy of Educational Objectives (Bloom, 1956)

Descriptions of the Major Categories in the Cognitive Domain

1. *Knowledge.* Knowledge is defined as the remembering of previously learned material. This may involve the recall of a wide range of material, from specific facts to complete theories, but all that is required is the bringing to mind of the appropriate information. Knowledge represents the lowest level of learning outcomes in the cognitive domain.

2. *Comprehension.* Comprehension is defined as the ability to grasp the meaning of material. This may be shown by translating material from one form to another (words to numbers), by interpreting material (explaining or summarizing), and by estimating future trends (predicting consequences or effects). These learning outcomes go one step beyond the simple remembering of material, and represent the lowest level of understanding.

3. *Application.* Application refers to the ability to use learned material in new and concrete situations. This may include the application of such things as rules, methods, concepts, principles, laws, and theories. Learning outcomes in this area require a higher level of understanding than those under comprehension.

4. *Analysis.* Analysis refers to the ability to break down material into its component parts so that its organizational structure may be understood. This may include the identification of the parts, analysis of the relationships between parts, and recognition of the organizational principles involved. Learning outcomes here represent a higher intellectual level than comprehension and application because they require an understanding of both the content and the structural form of the material.

5. *Synthesis.* Synthesis refers to the ability to put parts together to form a new whole. This may involve the production of a unique communication (theme or speech), a plan of operations (research proposal), or a set of abstract relations (scheme for classifying information). Learning outcomes in this area stress creative behaviors, with major emphasis on the formulation of *new* patterns or structures.

6. *Evaluation.* Evaluation is concerned with the ability to judge the value of material (statement, novel, poem, research report) for a given purpose. The judgments are to be based on definite criteria. These may be internal criteria (organization) or external criteria (relevance to the purpose) and the student may determine the criteria or be given them. Learning outcomes in this area are highest in the cognitive hierarchy because they contain elements of all of the other categories, plus conscious value judgments based on clearly defined criteria.

Figure 2
Major Categories in the Affective Domain
of the Taxonomy of Educational Objectives
(Krathwohl, 1964)

DESCRIPTIONS OF THE MAJOR CATEGORIES IN THE AFFECTIVE DOMAIN

1. *Receiving.* Receiving refers to the student's willingness to attend to particular phenomena or stimuli (classroom activities, textbook, music, etc.). From a teaching standpoint, it is concerned with getting, holding, and directing the student's attention. Learning outcomes in this area range from the simple awareness that a thing exists to selective attention on the part of the learner. Receiving represents the lowest level of learning outcomes in the affective domain.

2. *Responding.* Responding refers to active participation on the part of the student. At this level he not only attends to a particular phenomenon but also reacts to it in some way. Learning outcomes in this area may emphasize acquiescence in responding (reads assigned material), willingness to respond (voluntarily reads beyond assignment), or satisfaction in responding (reads for pleasure or enjoyment). The higher levels of this category include those instructional objectives that are commonly classified under "interest"; that is, those that stress the seeking out and enjoyment of particular activities.

3. *Valuing.* Valuing is concerned with the worth or value a student attaches to a particular object, phenomenon, or behavior. This ranges in degree from the more simple acceptance of value (desires to improve group skills) to the more complex level of commitment (assumes responsibility for the effective functioning of the group). Valuing is based on the internalization of a set of specified values, but clues to these values are expressed in the student's overt behavior. Learning outcomes in this area are concerned with behavior that is consistent and stable enough to make the value clearly identifiable. Instructional objectives that are commonly classified under "attitudes" and "appreciation" would fall into this category.

4. *Organization.* Organization is concerned with bringing together different values, resolving conflicts between them, and beginning the building of an internally consistent value system. Thus the emphasis is on comparing, relating, and synthesizing values. Learning outcomes may be concerned with the conceptualization of a value (recognizes the responsibility of each individual for improving human relations) or with the organization of a value system (develops a vocational plan that satisfies his need for both economic security and social service). Instructional objectives relating to the development of a philosophy of life would fall into this category.

5. *Characterization by a Value or Value Complex.* At this level of the affective domain, the individual has a value system that has controlled his behavior for a sufficiently long time for him to have developed a characteristic "life-style." Thus the behavior is pervasive, consistent, and predictable. Learning outcomes at this level cover a broad range of activities, but the major emphasis is on the fact that the behavior is typical or characteristic of the student. Instructional objectives that are concerned with the student's general patterns of adjustment (personal, social, emotional) would be appropriate here.

items were selected to represent the receiving, responding, valuing, and organization levels of the affective taxonomy for all five scale topics. Each of the five subscales contained eight attitude items, two items for each of the four levels of the affective taxonomy.

The instrument was evaluated by a panel of educational psychologists and a panel of health educators and was declared construct and content valid. Internal consistency for the cognitive scale, measured by the KR-20 at .70, and the value of 2.73 for the standard error of measurement were indications that the cognitive instrument was reliable. Cronbach reliability coefficients were computed for each subscale of the attitude scale; these ranged from .67 to .81. Based on subjective evaluation of the 40 attitude statements and the high reliability coefficients the affective instrument was deemed reliable.

Subjects

The subjects for this study included undergraduate students at a midwestern university during the fall (instrumentation phase) and spring (experimental phase) academic semesters, 1984–85. Approximately 90 students from two personal health education classes comprised the instrumentation phase. Subjects in the experimental group consisted of 396 students enrolled in all sections of personal health, who completed the survey questionnaire. Subjects in the control group included 110 students in English and math courses who agreed to respond to the knowledge and attitude questionnaire. English and math classes were chosen because of their similar ratio of freshmen and sophomores as well as males and females when compared to the composition of the personal health classes. Subjects in the control group were screened out if they had previously taken a formal college level course in personal health.

Owing to a small degree of attrition, coding errors, and incomplete questionnaires the experimental group was reduced from 430 to 396 subjects. The control group was also reduced in number from 117 to 110 subjects for final data analysis. Therefore, response rates for experimental and control groups totalled 92% and 94%, respectively.

Randomization of subjects was not considered a limitation for this investigation. All possible experimental subjects (i.e., all classes of the required-for-graduation personal health course for this particular spring semester) were included in the study, aside from the small number eliminated via attrition, coding errors, and incomplete questionnaires. However, subjects were randomly assigned to each class (experimental and control) via computer-assisted central registration procedures at this midwestern university.

Personal Health Education Intervention

The personal health classes utilized in this study were taught by four instructors from the same department within the university. All four instructors utilized the same organizational structure in regard to course objectives, outlines, required texts, evaluation scheme, and grading procedures. Audiovisuals, lectures, and supplemental handout materials were all standardized to enhance the consistency of the personal health education intervention for this study. The major focus of this basic health class was to increase student knowledge of, and value for, combatting the controllable risk factors associated with "life-style" related disease and disability. For this study nutrition-weight control, stress, exercise-rest, alcohol use, and smoking behavior were the major topics of the educational intervention.

Data Collection

The Knowledge and Attitude Survey was administered by the investigator for the sake of uniformity and to standardize test procedures. Pretests and posttests were administered on approximately the same calendar days for all experimental and control classes. Students were asked to cooperate by completing the Personal Health Knowledge and Attitude Questionnaire. Completion was *not* mandatory. Students were assured verbally that their individual responses would be kept confidential.

For matching pretests and posttests and for identification purposes, the students were asked to give their student identification (social security) number on the front page of the survey. These data collection procedures were followed for the pretest and posttest. All data from the Personal Health Knowledge and Attitude Questionnaire were transferred to computer optical scan sheets for statistical analysis. Subsequent analysis was performed by the investigator.

Data Analysis

The research design for this study was a repeated measures, pretest, posttest, experimental-control group design, with subjects matched across time. Data analysis was divided into two phases. Phase I pertained to the evaluation of cognitive and affective results of the required course in personal health. Statistical procedures for this phase utilized separate two-way ANOVAS (time × group) for the cognitive and affective taxonomic levels and also for total scores for these scales. Resultant *F*-ratios were tested at the .05 level of significance.

In the second phase, the relationship between cognitive and affective taxonomic outcomes of the required personal health course was examined. An analysis was performed in this phase on the affective subscale mean scores across four cognitive taxonomic levels, followed by four univariate F-test using Wilks Lambda (U-Statistic) to determine significant means differences. This mean score and post hoc analysis was performed on both the experimental and control group utilizing posttest data.

RESULTS

The results are based on data collected from the 506 subjects who completed the pretest and posttest questionnaires in the experimental phase of the study. The elapsed time between pre and post measurements was approximately four months (one semester).

Phase I: Cognitive and Affective Taxonomic Outcomes

Summarized results of the two-way ANOVAS (time = pre to post and group = experimental-control) computed on all four cognitive and affective taxonomic levels, and total scores for these scales are presented in Tables 1 and 2, respectively. The major concern in this first phase of data analysis was whether or not a treatment effect from the health education intervention occurred for cognition and affect. Therefore, only the significant ANOVA results are presented in Tables 1 and 2.

Cognitive results (Table 1) indicated a significant ($p < .01$) time × group interaction effect for the total cognitive scale scores. The experimental group (pre × = 41.26 and post × = 45.42) scored significantly higher than the control group (pre × = 41.8 and post × = 42.85) regarding personal health cognition over the course of one semester. Cognitive results also found significant ($p < .01$) time × group interactions (experimental control) for the Knowledge, Comprehension, and Application Taxonomic levels. However, analysis of variance for the Analysis-Synthesis Level found *no* significant time × group interaction (Table 1). This finding could be due, in part, to the difficulty of the Analysis-Synthesis level of cognition and also the possible lack of student experience in responding to items of this nature.

Examination of Table 2 indicated a significant ($p < .01$) time × group interaction affect for the total affective scale scores. As with cognition, the experimental group (pre × = 142.17 and post × = 148.36) had a significantly greater change in positive attitudes than did the control group (pre × = 141.99 and post × = 140.59) toward personal health from pretest to posttest.

TABLE 1

Summary Table of Significant Anova Main and Interaction Effects of
Cognitive Taxonomic Outcomes

	F Ratio	Significance Level
Total Cognitive Scale Scores		
Time	207.06	.01
Time × Group	404.02	.01
Knowledge Level		
Group	5.72	.05
Time	203.15	.01
Time × Group	42.02	.01
Comprehension Level		
Time	164.93	.01
Time × Group	27.33	.01
Application Level		
Group	11.48	.01
Time	104.06	.01
Time × Group	18.40	.01
Analysis-Synthesis		
Time	14.10	.01

This trend in significant ($p < .01$) time × group interaction (experimental control) was consistent for all affective taxonomic levels receiving, responding, valuing, and organization.

Results from Phase I indicated that a significant degree of cognitive learning and affective internalization had occurred for those students in the one semester personal health course. The next procedure was to evaluate the relationship between these cognitive and affective outcomes.

Phase II: Evaluation of the Relationship Between Cognitive and Affective Taxonomic Outcomes

The intent of this second phase was to determine the association between cognitive learning and affective internalization as a result of the personal health education course. In order to determine this, subjects had to be "grouped" or classified as belonging to one of the four cognitive levels of achievement. This was accomplished by computing average subscale scores for each student using posttest data.

TABLE 2
Summary Table of Significant Anova Main and Interaction Effects of
Affective Taxonomic Outcomes

	F Ratio	Significance Level
Total Affective Scale Scores		
Group	5.30	.05
Time	57.02	.01
Time × Group	29.65	.01
Receiving Level		
Group	5.62	.05
Time	31.29	.01
Time × Group	20.32	.01
Responding Level		
Time	20.15	.01
Time × Group	12.81	.01
Valuing Level		
Time	27.95	.01
Time × Group	18.05	.01
Organization Level		
Group	8.14	.01
Time	46.95	.01
Time × Group	14.69	.01

The number of correct responses for each subscale was divided by the number of items in each subscale, that is, 8 of 10 = 80% achievement for a given subscale. It was determined by the investigators that an achievement of 60% or better (6 correct responses out of 10 items) would be the criteria for classification of a subject by taxonomic level. For example, if a subject received a 60% rating at the knowledge level, a 60% rating at the comprehension level, a 60% rating at the application level, and a 40% rating at the Analysis-Synthesis level, he or she would belong to the application group or level of achievement. As a result of the above classification scheme there were 120 students classified at the Knowledge Level, 72 at the Comprehension Level, 132 at the Application Level, and 64 at the Analysis/Synthesis Level.

The affective domain level scores by level of cognitive achievement are presented in Table 3. The average affective level scores presented in the first

TABLE 3
Analysis of Affective Domain Level Scores Across Four Cognitive Domain Levels of Achievement

Students Achieving At:	Average Affective Level Scores	Receiving X̄ Scores	Responding X̄ Scores	Valuing X̄ Scores	Organization X̄ Scores
KNOWLEDGE LEVEL (*n*=120)	36.6	38.44	33.95	39.23	34.67
COMPREHENSION LEVEL (*n*=72)	37.1	39.79	34.36	39.14	35.24
APPLICATION LEVEL (*n*=132)	37.4	39.93	35.00	39.57	34.92
ANALYSIS -SYNTHESIS LEVEL (*n*=64)	38.6	41.07	35.40	41.55	36.31

column of Table 3 indicate that the students classified in higher cognitive levels received, on the average, higher affective level scores than did students classified in lower cognitive levels. These progressive differences failed to reach statistical significance ($p < .07$).

However, within each affective level experimental students scored progressively higher at each cognitive level (e.g., within each affective level, students classified at the Analysis-Synthesis level had the highest scores followed in order by the students classified at the Application Level, Comprehension Level, and Knowledge Level). To determine the significance of the differences found between Cognitive Levels, four univariate *F*-tests using Wilks Lamda (U-statistic) were performed on each of the four affective domain level scores. The results of these analyses, presented in Table 4, indicate the statistical significance ($p < .05$) of this trend for the Receiving and Valuing Domain Scores.

As a comparative measure the same analyses were performed on the subjects in the control group. These analyses indicated that affective mean scores across the four cognitive taxonomic levels were scattered and showed no pattern of performance from lower to higher taxonomic levels. Post hoc analysis also indicated no significant differences between group or taxonomic mean scores.

TABLE 4

Univariate *F*-Tests Using Wilks Lambda (U-Statistic) for the Affective
Taxonomic Subscales Experimental Group Mean Scores

Taxonomic Subscale	Wilks Lambda	F	Significance
Receiving	.974	3.25	.02*
Responding	.989	1.21	.31
Valuing	.966	3.82	.01**
Organization	.990	1.56	.33

*Significant at/or beyond the .05 level
**Significant at/or beyond the .01 level

CONCLUSIONS

Findings of this study demonstrated that a relationship does exist between cognitive learning and affective internalization, and that this relationship is operative at the lower levels as well as the higher levels of the taxonomy. Data presented in Table 3 demonstrated that affective change increased in a consistent trend as the level of cognitive difficulty increased. This overall linear pattern of higher affective performance at higher levels of cognition in this study also supported the theory that the structure of the cognitive and affective taxonomies are hierarchical in nature.

The significant findings for the receiving and valuing levels (Table 4) are difficult to interpret. Perhaps in this particular study the receiving and valuing levels had the greatest discriminatory power. The organization level represents an individual's development and consistent use of a life plan and philosophy of healthy living. Perhaps it is too much to expect from college freshmen and sophomores to have, from a one-semester required course in personal health, a well-defined plan for a healthy adult life-style as well as a corresponding philosophy of life relating to positive health behavior.

In reexamination of some of the responding level items, it is possible that positive responses to these actually represent a higher level than valuing. To illustrate, the statement, "I have gone to lectures, workshops, classes, and other sources of information to find out more about stress management," was assigned to the Responding category; but because this statement is related to the actual behavior of seeking additional information, which may or may not be readily available on campus, it is entirely possible that positive responses to this statement actually represent a *higher* level than Responding. The inherent value of these results in health education is that cognitive learning and affective internalization take place in a "building block" manner, and that both domains have in their lower levels simple, concrete learning behaviors, which serve as foundations for more complex learning behavior. These results suggest that students in health education courses need basic information, but also need to be challenged to apply, analyze, and synthesize health information as it relates to higher affective performance and ultimately the development of healthy life-styles.

Discussion: The Relationship Between Health Knowledge, Attitudes, and Behavior

The most critical assumption underlying behavioral and life-style change is the fundamental principle of health education: that individuals, families, small groups, and communities can be taught to assume responsibility for their health and that this assumption of responsibility, in turn, brings about changes in their health behaviors and lifestyles (Bates & Winder, 1984). Green, Kreuter, Deeds, and Partridge (1980) define health education as "any combination of learning experiences designed to facilitate voluntary adaptions of behavior conducive to health" (p. 7).

The mission of Health Education, as suggested by Bedworth and Bedworth (1978) is to provide the individual with the ingredients necessary for more effective living. Health goals are related to these ingredients. A health goal, therefore, is the predetermined purpose of health learning experiences.

Changes in knowledge and attitudes are thus acknowledged as precursors to appropriate health behavior. Although increases in knowledge and development of positive attitudes may be deemed as desirable outcomes in personal health education programs, these changes alone will not guarantee subsequent improvement in personal health behavior. The relationship between knowledge, attitudes, and behavior is quite complex. Iverson and Portnoy (1977) view the knowledge/attitude/behavior triad in the following manner:

> The assumed role of educational programs in behavior change is to directly increase knowledge and indirectly initiate attitude and behavior changes. Knowledge then functions as a direct and indirect stimulus for change in attitudes and a direct change agent for behavior. Knowledge will function as a direct change agent for attitudes far more frequently than it will for behaviors. Attitudes are direct and indirect change agents for behavior. Once a behavior is altered there is, in many instances, a direct feedback mechanism which alters the appropriate attitudes in such a manner as to reinforce the new behavior. (p.   )

Knowledge, attitudes, and behavior are then viewed as *interacting* variables with complex feedback mechanisms. Green et al. (1980) also contend
that the association between knowledge and health is more than philosophic.
They suggest that knowledge helps to increase decision-making abilities and
skills that *may* contribute to positive health behavior.

Educational programs generally have the effect of increasing knowledge
levels in specific areas such as smoking, contraception, or nutritional health.
The increased knowledge may then initiate direct or indirect changes in
attitudes. These changes in knowledge and attitude may then precipitate
behavioral changes.

Findings from this study did identify the overall pattern of higher affective
performance at higher levels of cognition for those subjects exposed to the
health education intervention (the required course in personal health).
According to the theory proposed in the Taxonomy of Educational Objectives, performance at the Valuing and Organization levels of the Affective
Domain (see figures 1 and 2) is indicative of appropriate or positive health
behavior. In view of the fact that these findings were self-reported, they do
point out the potential for effective, challenging, and well-planned health
education interventions, to have a positive impact on health behavior via
modification, maintenance, and change.

Again, affect, cognition, and behavior should be viewed as *interacting*
variables with complex feedback loops and mechanisms. An increase in affect
can increase cognitive learning and vice versa. Because these variables are
interacting, learning in health education should consider the theoretical
framework of the Taxonomy of Educational Objectives as one important
avenue to learning that can lead to positive health behavior.

In summary, there is no direct association among cognitive learning,
affective internalization, and health behavior. However, the results of this
study do suggest that an increase in cognition about health and the
acquisition of positive attitudes toward one's health, may contribute to
motivating and influencing positive health behaviors.

IMPLICATIONS

Findings of this study suggest the following implications for personal health
and also for the field of health education in general.

Utilizing the Taxonomy of Educational Objectives
as a Theoretical Framework

This study would not have been possible without the hierarchical structure of
the Cognitive and Affective Domains of the Taxonomy of Educational

Objectives. This earlier work by Bloom (1956) and Krathohl (1964) was most instrumental in assisting the four personal health instructors in operationalizing their educational objectives and the standardized interventions to meet them. The Taxonomy significantly aided in developing the Table of Specifications for designing both the Knowledge and Attitude scales used to measure the results of Phase I and II. Most noteworthy here is the ability of the taxonomy to assist in developing scale items that measure more complex learning. The recall of factual information or simple receiving of value statements would seldom require a sophisticated structure such as the Cognitive and Affective Domains of the Taxonomy of Educational Objectives.

Unfortunately, as indicated by Bloom (1984) most of the teacher made tests today in the United States are largely tests of remembered information. After the sale of over one million copies of the Taxonomy of Educational Objectives—Cognitive Domain (Bloom, 1956) and over a quarter of a century of use of this domain in preservice and inservice teacher training, it is estimated that 90% of test questions that U.S. school students are expected to answer today still deal with little more than information. Our instructional material, our classroom teaching methods, and our testing methods rarely rise above the lowest level of the Taxonomy, knowledge, or the pursuit of trivia.

Measuring Specificity of Attitude Change

In regard to health behavior as a desired outcome of Health Education programs, use of the Taxonomy should be continued. Stainbrook and Green (1982) feel that the one constant finding on which health education researchers can rely is that attitudes predict behavior better as the specificity of the attitude increases. The use of the Taxonomy (affective domain) is one method of disecting specificity of attitude based on a hierarchical model moving from simple to complex. Examination of Figure 2 depicts the ability of the major categories of the Affective Domain of the Taxonomy of Educational Objectives to measure attitude change by specific taxonomic level. The major categories can be disected even further depending upon the nature, limitations, and major objectives of a given investigation. For those researchers interested in breaking down the Cognitive and Affective Domains, securing a copy of Handbooks I and II by Bloom (1956) and Krathwohl (1964) is recommended.

Generalized Application of the Taxonomy to Health Education Programs

Comprehensive school health education programs offered in grades K–12 could make use of the Taxonomy in planning, implementing, and evaluating their curricula. The building block nature of the model would be most applicable for these school-based programs with lower grade levels mastering lower hierarchical levels before being introduced to the higher levels.

A hierarchical model of learning such as the Taxonomy of Educational Objectives should be utilized in planning, implementing, and evaluating other health education programs. The usefulness of this model, as evidenced by this study, in evaluating the relationship between cognitive, affective outcomes should be utilized in such programs as smoking cessation, weight management, contraceptive use, stress management, and seat belt use, where positive behavior change is the desired outcome.

A table of specifications could be designed, utilizing both the affective and cognitive domains, as a framework for any aspect of a health education and/or health promotion program. These include the following examples:

1. Instructional objectives at each desired level of the Taxonomy can be determined.
2. The amount of instructional time devoted to each level of cognitive learning and affect can be planned.
3. Lecture content to be utilized at each taxonomic level can be planned for and classified.
4. Learning strategies and creative instructional techniques by both level of cognition and degree of affective internalization can be planned and implemented.
5. Evaluation schemes and techniques can be designed by taxonomic level. Emphasis can be placed on the level of learning expected, depending upon variables such as, target group, age, type of intervention/ instruction and learning objectives.
6. Multiple choice, matching, fill-in-the-blank, true-false, and essay test questions can all be designed via the principles of the Taxonomy of Educational Objectives.

It is recommended that both domains of this theoretical framework be utilized effectively. A close relationship exists between the cognitive and affective domains of the Taxonomy, they are parallel in nature and there is an intimate relationship between cognitive and affective learning. This relationship is operative at the knowledge-receiving levels as well as the analysis/synthesis-organization levels.

Health educators and researchers are advised to secure a copy of both Handbooks I and II of the Taxonomy of Educational Objectives. These publications explain in detail the diverse applicability of this theoretical structure to educational efforts (Bloom, 1956; Krathwohl, 1964).

Teaching to the Acquisition of Higher Mental Processes

The most significant suggestion this investigation offers, is for health education curriculum, instructional objectives, methodologies, and evaluation (testing) procedures to be designed at all levels of the Taxonomy, especially the higher levels of the cognitive and affective domains. Results from the second phase of data analysis indicated an overall pattern of higher affective performance at higher levels of cognition. Students in the required personal health course who performed at the analysis-synthesis level of cognition were more likely to perform at the organization level of affect. The implication is that by teaching to the higher levels of cognition a health educator may also be developing positive attitudes and vice versa. Though the more common route is from the cognitive to the affective, it is quite possible that teaching to the higher levels of affect may motivate the learner to achieve at higher levels of cognition. Health educators may wish to acknowledge these findings since the goals of Health Education are to provide information, develop positive health attitudes, and, ultimately, modify or change health behaviors. Therefore, greater emphasis should be placed on problem solving, application of principles, analytical skills, and creativity. This implies that all of these methods should be reflected in the health education materials of instruction, the learning and teaching processes used, and the questions and problems used in the formative testing and final summative evaluations.

The acquisition of higher mental processes may also enable the student to relate his or her learning to the various problems encountered in day-to-day living. These abilities—problem solving, application of principles, analytical skills, and creativity—should also be stressed because, according to Bloom (1984), they are retained and used long after the individual has forgotten the detailed specifics of the subject matter taught in class. These abilities are regarded as one set of essential characteristics needed to cope with a rapidly changing world.

REFERENCES

Bates, I. J., & Winder, A. E. (1984). *Introduction To Health Education.* Palo Alto, CA: Mayfield.
Bedworth, D. A., & Bedworth, A. E. (1978). *Health Education: A Process for Human Effectiveness.* New York: Harper and Row.
Bloom, B. S. (1956). *Taxonomy of Educational Objectives: Handbooks I: Cognitive Domain.* New York: David McKay Company, Inc.

Bloom, B. S. (1984). The 2 sigma problem: The search for methods of group instruction as effective as one to one tutoring. *Educational Researcher, 13*(6), 4–15.

Green, K., Kreuter, M., Deeds, S., & Partridge, K. (1980). *Health Education Planning—A Diagnostic Approach.* Palo Alto, CA: Mayfield Publishing Company.

Iverson, D., & Portnoy, B. (1977). Reassessment of the knowledge/attitude/behavior triad. *Health Education, 8,* 31–34.

Krathwohl, D. R. (1964). *Taxonomy of Educational Objectives: Handbook II: Affective Domain.* New York: David McKay Company, Inc.

Lewy, A. (1968, Spring). The Empirical validity of major properties of a taxonomy of affective educational objective. *Journal of Experimental Education, 36*(3)

Stainbrook, G., & Green, L. W. (1982). Behavior and Behaviorism in Health Education. *Health Education, 13,* 14–19.

Stroker, H. W., & Kroop, R. P. (1964). Measurement of Cognitive Process. *Journal of Educational Measurement, 1,* 39–42.

4

HEALTH EDUCATION TEXTBOOKS: A HALF-CENTURY OF PUBLIC SCHOOL USE, 1905–1955

Richard K. Means

One purpose of the study was the inclusion of a representative listing of health education textbooks from 1905–55. Investigation indicated that no such compilation and analysis heretofore appeared in print. The 297 textbooks included in the study are included as an appendix.

A second, and more important purpose encompassed a half-century analysis of the titles and "inferred" content included in health education textbooks during the period. Two comprehensive tables are included to provide a consolidation of these results.

A corraborative historical analysis also is provided to help substantiate the findings. This carefully documented analysis served to help trace curriculum development in the field. The results of this evaluation of school health textbooks throughout the period in the field should be of value to historical researchers.

REVIEW OF LITERATURE

Prior to 1905

A fairly extensive introduction to health education textbooks and text-book-type materials seems appropriate. This is due, in part, to the fact that very little attention to the subject previously has been cited in published form.

Perhaps earliest references to such materials evolved around the turn of the nineteenth century. One important development was traced by Rogers (1940). He asserted that:

It was from a small province of Germany that we derived our beginings in formal
health instruction, and the first course of study to be used by teachers and pupils,
issued in 1792, was received with enthusiasm. . . . It was reprinted in New York in
1798 and was still alive as late as 1882. (p. 9)

This document had worldwide acceptance. Within 10 years of its
publication 150,000 copies had been sold. It was translated into English,
Swedish, Bohemian, Dutch, Slavonic, Italian, Icelandic, Polish, French, and
Lettish.

Many early textbooks in health education were written by physicians in
other countries, according to Means (1975, p. 67). These slowly flowed from
Europe into the United States in the 1800s.

Around the turn of the eighteenth century the Reverend Mason Weems
printed and promoted a health book in the United States. The text evolved
into six editions and was primarily intended for use by adults. It was reported
to have been enhanced by a letter of recommendation from George
Washington.

Rogers (1940), reported that "school health texts had been published since
the earliest days of public schools" (p. 1). A footnote to this reference
specified that the earliest might have been in the year 1837 related to the
common school movement in Massachusetts. As common education grew
and the health education curriculum expanded, an increasing number of
textbooks were published.

According to Rogers (1940), "By 1880 there were at least 36 textbooks in
use" (p. 11), and among them a work approved and "enriched" by the
president of a state medical association and by at least sixteen school
principals and teachers of science. Kleinschmidt (1950, p. 38) indicated that
one of the most widely utilized earlier books was the *Health Primer*.

During the same approximate period, considerable textbook influence was
felt as a result of the activities of the Women's Christian Temperance Union,
founded in 1874. At this time hygiene and physiology courses were much in
evidence and often were compulsory. The W.C.T.U. was responsible for the
passing of legislation related to such instruction. This was described as
follows by Rogers (1930):

No wave of legislation having to do with school hygiene and sanitation has so
swept the country as that accompanying the temperance movement. Every state
passed a law requiring instruction in regard to the effects of alcohol and
narcotics; while for the territories a law to the same effect was established by act
of Congress. (p. 1)

Some laws actually specified the amount of space or number of pages to be devoted to the subject in books adopted for such instruction. The earliest evidence of health education in the schools were these courses in anatomy, physiology, and hygiene, or combinations of the three areas. The foregoing emphases continued from the end of the nineteenth century until well into the 1900s. By the beginning of the period covered by this investigation (1905) other topics were emerging.

From 1905–55

A number of studies were conducted related to textbook analysis during the years from 1905–55. Most of these, however, were quite limited in scope. Collectively, the studies ranged from an evaluation of 3 to 36 textbooks.

At the elementary and junior high school level specifically, four textbook studies were uncovered. Bobbit (1925) included textbooks along with an evaluation of newspapers and magazines in an attempt to identify the objectives of health education through an evaluation of health topics. Merrill (1949) assessed 36 selected textbooks in a process of determining concepts of healthful living of value in contributing to general education.

A dissertation by Foster (1953) provided an analysis of health information in 36 textbooks for grades one through six. Ludwig (1953) conducted a comparative investigation of 14 health textbooks for grades seven and eight.

Other studies included elementary and junior high school textbooks, but only as a part of a broader appraisal. Strang (1926) conducted an analysis of 14 textbooks along with selected courses of study and several other publications to determine subject matter emphasis. A year later, Meir (1927) identified health content covered in seven general science textbooks.

Means (1928) evaluated 34 textbooks in physiology. A year later, Chappelear (1929) did the same for health subject matter in 20 natural sciences books. Hewlett (1935) studied the overlap of content in health education, general science, and biology textbooks using 12 different books.

Three textbook investigations were conducted in the 1940s. Van Heuvelen (1940) assessed health education subject matter found in 14 high school chemistry textbooks. A year later, Hurd (1941) evaluated 10 general science textbooks with the same purpose.

Staton (1948) utilized 10 health textbooks and 36 issues of *Hygeia* magazine in an effort to identify fundamental health concepts. These were evaluated on the basis of the importance for general education at the secondary level.

Two additional studies were completed through the period of this investigation, both in 1953. Kilander, Hein, and Mitchell (1953) reported on the accuracy of health textbook content in the *Journal of School Health*.

Worick (1953) developed his dissertation around an analysis of three state-adopted biology textbooks. These were appraised in their application to health education.

PROCEDURES FOLLOWED

The collection of data for the study consisted of the location of school health textbooks published for the 50-year period from 1905 to 1955. Basic sources of information included the author's personal historical collection; references available at Auburn University, at Teachers College, Columbia University; those located at the Library of Congress in Washington, D.C.; and other general library resources.

A total of 297 books comprised the final list. Full bibliographical information was recorded for each reference. These were organized into three grade levels—elementary, junior high school, and high school. A topical list was then compiled of descriptive terms found in each textbook title. Several dozen such terms comprised an initial list, which was reduced to 11 topics on the basis of a minimum of at least three citations over the years.

The data obtained were organized by decades over the 50-year period both by grade level and in a combined fashion for analysis. These data are presented in tabular form in the analysis section of the report.

SCHOOL HEALTH TEXTBOOKS, 1905–55

An investigation was conducted of school health textbooks, grades 1 through 12, for the years 1905–55. A total of 297 textbooks comprised the final listing. These were divided into those intended for the elementary school level ($n =$ 104), the junior high school ($n = 84$), and the high school level ($n = 109$). This was not a complete list, but it is considered "more than representative" of the textbooks published for health instruction during the 50-year period.

Health Textbook Analysis

In order to provide a historical perspective, the 297 textbooks listed were evaluated on the basis of major topical headings appearing in the titles. This analysis was conducted on a decade-by-decade basis for the 50-year period. These data were then organized into two descriptive tables.

In Table 1 overall findings were tabulated. A list of topics indicated in textbook titles is presented alphabetically in the left-hand column. The least

TABLE 1

Health Titles in Textbooks (1905–55)

Topics in Title	Elementary 104 Textbooks					Jr. H. S. 84 Textbooks					High School 109 Textbooks					Total*
	1905 –15	1916 –25	1926 –35	1936 –45	1946 –55	1905 –15	1916 –25	1926 –35	1936 –45	1946 –55	1905 –15	1916 –25	1926 –35	1936 –45	1946 –55	
Anatomy	1	0	0	0	0	2	0	0	0	0	2	1	0	0	0	6
Cleanliness	1	1	0	0	0	0	0	0	1	0	0	0	0	0	0	3
Growth	0	0	1	3	2	0	0	0	0	0	0	0	1	0	1	8
Health	7	10	15	20	7	4	10	11	16	8	3	7	18	27	10	173
Human Body	1	1	2	0	0	5	4	3	3	1	1	1	3	3	1	29
Hygiene	7	9	4	1	0	5	7	0	0	0	12	6	2	0	1	54
Keeping Well	1	0	5	8	1	1	2	5	5	2	2	6	4	5	4	51
Physiology	6	6	3	0	0	7	5	0	0	0	14	6	2	1	0	50
Public Health	0	0	0	0	0	0	1	2	0	0	0	1	3	2	0	9
Safety	0	0	0	1	0	0	1	0	1	0	0	0	0	4	2	9
Sanitation	3	2	0	0	0	0	0	0	0	0	1	3	0	0	0	9
Total*	27	29	30	33	10	24	30	21	26	11	35	31	33	42	19	401

*Total exceeds the number of books surveyed (297) because several topics were sometimes included in a single title.

number of times a topic was cited was 3 (cleanliness), and the most frequent
was 173 times (health). Next in order of frequency were hygiene (54),
keeping well (51), and physiology (50).

Anatomy, physiology, and hygiene combined provided a total citation of
110. These were common topics particularly in the early decades of the
period. Because several topics were sometimes included in a single title, the
total number of citations (401) exceeds the number of books (297).

Table 1 also was organized to depict the three grade levels covered by the
study. Elementary school textbooks numbered 104, junior high, 84, and high
school books, 109. Textbooks for each level were correlated by topic in the
decade-by-decade format. Titles included for each decade included: 1905–15
(86), 1916–25 (90), 1926–35 (84), 1936–45 (101) and 1946–55 (40). The table
provides a compact and easy reference for the overall project.

A composite of textbook titles for the period is presented in Table 2. The
topics included remained the same, and a decade-by-decade analysis again
was provided. However, each column from 1905–55 represented a synop-
sis of the textbooks without specific grade level designation. For example,
24 textbooks with "hygiene" in the title were identified in the sample
from 1905–15. These included elementary, junior high, and high school
books.

TABLE 2
Composite of Textbook Titles, 1905–55
(Combined elementary, junior high, and high school textbooks)

Topics in Title	1905–15	1926–25	1926–35	1936–45	1946–55	Total*
Anatomy	5	1	0	0	0	6
Cleanliness	1	1	0	1	0	3
Growth	0	0	2	3	3	8
Health	14	27	44	63	25	173
Human Body	7	6	8	6	2	29
Hygiene	24	22	6	1	1	54
Keeping Well	4	8	14	18	7	51
Physiology	27	17	5	1	0	50
Public Health	0	2	5	2	0	9
Safety	0	1	0	6	2	9
Sanitation	4	5	0	0	0	9
TOTAL	86	90	84	101	40	401

*Total exceeds the number of books surveyed (297) because several topics were sometimes
included in a single title.

Findings and Corroborative Studies

A further assessment of the tables, especially Table 2, would indicate some important findings. These are summarized as follows, along with collaborating historical research.

1. Physiology as a topic in textbook titles led all others for the decade 1905–15 ($n = 27$); it was third ($n = 17$) in the next decade, but then dropped drastically. Only a single health education textbook title included physiology from 1936 on.

Of significance was the relative importance of physiology up until about 1930. The historical influence most significant in this evolvement was the development of the temperance movement, basically involving instruction regarding the effects of alcohol, tobacco, and narcotics, and previously reported.

The influence on textbooks of the period (1880 into the early 1900s) was identified by Rogers (1930). He pointed out that "such teaching belonged as part and parcel of the larger subjects of physiology and hygiene and these more general branches are required without limitation as to content by 40 states" (p. 2).

A series of bibliographies was published by Affleck (1910). This furnished a broad perspective of the literature during this early period. The information presented was very much in keeping with the textbook titles cited in the tables.

2. Hygiene as a topic closely followed the same pattern as physiology. It was second on the list ($n = 24$) for the first decade, second ($n = 22$) for the next decade, and then decreased rapidly. Only two books with hygiene in the title were published since 1936.

Hygiene as a topic was often included along with physiology in earlier references. It was frequently cited before the term health education came into usage around World War II.

An impetus to hygiene was provided by the periodical *American Journal of School Hygiene*. This was initially issued in January of 1917. In 1922, the name was changed to the *School Hygiene Review*. Basically, these publications helped to stimulate hygiene as a subject. These were reported by Averill (1922).

3. Anatomy, cleanliness, and sanitation as cited topics appeared basically in the decades between 1905–25 (combined $n = 17$). Only a single citation was noted for any of the three areas after 1925.

Anatomy as a topic often accompanied physiology and sometimes hygiene as a subject area in health education. Cleanliness and sanitation, on the other hand, were quite separate.

A stimulus for emphasis on these latter topics was undoubtedly derived from the formation of the Cleanliness Institute. This was a group composed of soap and glycerin manufacturers. According to Mitchell (1960, p. 3), they merged together to promote their products through health education.

4. Health as a topic was by far the most frequently cited for the 50 year period ($n = 173$). For the decade, 1905–15, however, it ranked only third ($n = 14$). From that point up to the end of the period, it led all others. From 1926–55, health accounted for over 50% of the citations.

Little historical documentation should be needed related to this particular finding. In the earliest decade of the study, it received only limited mention. This was due to the organizational patterns and printed materials reflecting the temperance subjects and instruction provided specifically through courses in anatomy, physiology, and hygiene.

5. Safety, public health, and growth were topics of apparent later interest. None of the three were mentioned in the·initial decade. Safety and growth had most frequent mention since 1936.

Public health as a topic in textbooks emerged somewhat midway in the period covered by the study and has reemerged in more recent years. Growth was initially mentioned twice as a topic in the 1925–36 decade, and three times in each of the subsequent two decades.

Safety as a topic enjoyed a somewhat separate evolution of its own. In certain ways it paralleled that of health education, although appearing somewhat later.

An early leader in the effort to put safety education into the curriculum described several developments that had an eventual impact on textbooks during the period. Stack (1960) outlined these as follows:

> One of the most notable developments in safety education, following World War I, was the conduct of some of the most significant research studies. . . . The first laws relating to instruction in safety education had to do with specific topics such as fire prevention, traffic safety, and bicycle safety. . . . The most recent wave of legislation—that for safety education—was set in motion by the speeding automobile. (pp. 2, 8)

6. The topics of the human body and "keeping well" were relatively consistently cited throughout the period. Keeping well was a common citation for the two decades from 1926–45 with 32 textbooks identified.

These two rather general topics of keeping well and the human body followed the logical pattern associated with evolutionary developments in anatomy, physiology, and hygiene. Citations support the greatest emphasis during the middle decades of the investigation.

CONCLUDING STATEMENT

It is apparent that basic textbooks in health education closely followed developments in legislative action and curriculum reform. This began with an early emphasis on anatomy, physiology, and hygiene. These were topics that in turn reflected a focus on the temperance subjects.

The topics of keeping well and health were rather consistently cited throughout the period but especially prominent in the middle decades of the period. More recent additions to textbook titles were the topics of growth, public health, and safety.

In certain instances, school health education publications lagged slightly behind evolving developments in the field. Overall, however, the textbooks seemed to reflect relatively quickly major changes in the field.

The evolution of health education as a field continues to be written. Only through the "bits and pieces" of continuing historical research will a substantive heritage be achieved. It is hoped that this study might provide yet another dimension toward the realization of a more definitive evaluation of health education.

REFERENCES

Affleck, G. (1910). Bibliography of Physical Training. *American Physical Education Review, 15*, 193–209.

Averill, L. (1922). The Progress of Hygiene. *School Hygiene Review, 6*, 37–46.

Bobbit, F. (1925). Discovering the Objectives of Health Education: Study of Health Topics in Newspapers, Magazines and Textbooks. *Elementary School Journal, 25*, 756–60.

Chappelear, C. (1929). *Health Subject Matter in Natural Sciences*. Doctoral dissertation, Teachers College, Columbia University, New York.

Foster, R. (1953). *An Analysis of the Type and Quantity of Health Information in Selected Health Education Textbooks For Grades One Through Six*. Doctoral dissertation, Indiana University, Bloomington.

Hewlett, A. (1935). *The Overlap of Health Education Subject Matter in Health Education, General Science, and Biology Textbooks*. Master's Thesis, State University of Iowa, Iowa City.

Hurd, J. (1941). An Evaluation of Certain General Science Textbooks on the Basis of Their Contribution to Health Education. *Science Education, 25*, 327–30.

Kilander, H., Hein, F., & Mitchell, H. (1953). The Accuracy of Health Content of School Textbooks. *Journal School Health, 23*, 216–22.

Kleinschmidt, H. (1950). Half-Century Mark: Health Education. *Today's Health, 28*, 38.

Ludwig, D. (1953). *An Analysis of the Health Information in Selected Health Education Textbooks for Grades Seven and Eight*. Doctoral dissertation, Indiana University, Bloomington.

Means, H. (1928). *An Analysis of Thirty Four Textbooks in Physiology*. Master's Thesis, Bloomington: Indiana University.

Means, R. (1975). *Historical Perspectives on School Health*. Thorofare, NJ: Charles B. Slack, Inc.

Meir, L. (1927). *Health Material in Science Textbooks*. Doctoral dissertation, Teachers College, Columbia University, New York.

Merrill, C. (1949). *A Determination of Concepts of Healthful Living Which Are of Fundamental Value in Contributing to the General Education of Elementary School Pupils.* Doctoral dissertation, Boston University, Boston.

Mitchell, H. (1960). Unpublished manuscript of personal interview. Laytonsville, MD.

Rogers, J. (1940). *Our Heritage in Health Education.* Unpublished manuscript.

Rogers, J. (1930). *State-Wide Trends in School Hygiene and Physical Education.* U.S. Department of the Interior, Office of Education, Pamphlet No. 5 (rev.), Washington, DC: Government Printing Office.

Stack, H. (1960). Unpublished manuscript of personal interview.

Strang, R. (1926). *Subject Matter in Health Education.* Doctoral dissertation, Teachers College, Columbia University, New York.

Staton, W. (1948). *A Determination of Fundamental Concepts of Healthful Living and Their Relative Importance for General Education at the Secondary Level,* Doctoral dissertation, Boston University, Boston.

Van Heuvelen, W. (1940). *Health Education Subject Matter Found in High School Chemistry Textbooks.* Master's thesis, University of Colorado, Boulder.

Worick, W. (1953). *An Analysis of the Contribution of Biology Instruction to Health Education.* Doctoral Dissertation, Indiana University, Bloomington.

APPENDIX A

Elementary School Textbooks
1905–1955

Author	Publisher	Title	Date	Grade
Coleman, Walter M.	The Macmillan Company	Lessons in Hygienic Physiology	1905	Elem.
Brown, B. M.	D. C. Heath and Company	Good Health for Boys & Girls	1906	Elem.
Stowell, C. H.	Silver, Burdett and Company	A Primer of Health-I	1906	U. El.
Stowell, C. H.	Silver, Burdett and Company	A Primer of Health-II	1906	L. El.
Blaisdell, A. F.	Ginn and Company	How to Keep Well	1907	Elem.
Krohn, William O.	D. Appleton and Company	Graded Lessons in Hygiene	1908	Elem.
Jewett, F. G.	Ginn and Company	The Body at Work	1909	Elem.
Conn, Herbert W.	Silver, Burdett and Company	Elementary Physiology and Hygiene	1910	U. El.
Davison, Alvin	American Book Company	Health Lessons Book I	1910	L. El.
Davison, Alvin	American Book Company	Health Lessons: Book II	1910	U. El.
Ritchie, John W.	World Book Company	Sanitation and Physiology	1910	Elem.
Ritchie, John W.	W. W. Shannon	Primer of Hygiene	1911	Elem.
Brown, B. M.	D. C. Heath and Company	Health in Home and Town	1912	U. El.
Krohn, William O.	D. Appleton and Company	Graded Lessons in Physiology and Hygiene	1912	L. El.
Overton, Frank	American Book Company	General Hygiene	1913	Elem.
Ritchie, John W.	World Book Company	Primer of Hygiene and Sanitation	1913	Elem.

Author	Publisher	Title	Date	Grade
Emerson, C. P., & Betts, G. H.	Bobbs-Merrill Company	Physiology and Hygiene	1915	Elem.
O'Shea, M. V., & Kellogg, J. H.	The Macmillan Company	Health and Cleanliness	1915	Elem.
Ritchie, J. W.	World Book Company	Primer: Sanitation, Physiology	1915	U. El.
Conn, H. W.	Silver, Burdett and Company	Physiology and Health: Book I	1916	L. El.
Jewett, F. G.	Ginn and Company	Physiology, Hygiene & Sanitation	1916	Elem.
Emerson, Charles P.	Bobbs-Merrill Company	Hygiene and Health	1919	Elem.
Heizer, W. Lucien	C. T. Dearing Printing Company	Physiology, Hygiene and Sanitation	1919	Elem.
Ritchie, John W.	World Book Company	New Primer of Hygiene	1919	Elem.
Conn, H. W., & Holt, C. M.	Silver, Burdett and Company	Physiology and Health: I	1920	L. El.
Conn, H. W., & Holt, C. M.	Silver, Burdett and Company	Physiology and Health: II	1920	U. El.
Ritchie, John W.	World Book Company	Human Physiology	1920	Elem.
Winslow, C-E, A.	Charles E. Merrill	Healthy Living: Book I	1920	Elem.
Emerson, C. P., & Betts, G. H.	Bobbs-Merrill Company	Hygiene and Health	1921	Elem.
Cobb, W. F.	World Book Company	Graded Outlines in Hygiene I	1922	Elem.
Dore, Francis J.	Joseph F. Wagner, Incorporated	Health and Happiness	1922	Elem.
Chubb, E. M.	Longman's, Green and Company	Our Bodies and How They Work	1923	Elem.
Cuzzort, B., & Trask, J. W.	D. C. Heath and Company	Health and Health Practices	1923	Elem.
O'Shea, M. V. & Kellogg, J. H.	The Macmillan Company	Building Health Habits	1923	Elem.
Trask, J. W.	D. C. Heath and Company	Primer of Personal Hygiene	1923	M. El.
Bigelow, M. A., & Broadhurst, J.	Silver, Burdett, & Company	Health for Every Day	1924	Elem.
Cobb, W. F.	World Book Company	Graded Outlines in Hygiene II	1924	Elem.
Davison, Alvin	American Book Company	Health Lessons Revised II	1924	Elem.
Davison, Alvin	American Book Company	Health Lessons Revised I	1924	Elem.
O'Shea, M. V., & Kellogg, J. H.	The Macmillan Company	Health and Cleanliness	1924	Elem.

Author	Publisher	Title	Date	Grade
Winslow, C-E. A.	Charles E. Merrill	Health Living: Book II	1924	U. El.
Burkard, W. E., et. al.	Lyons and Carnahan	Health Habits by Practice	1925	Elem.
Burkard, W. E., et. al.	Lyons and Carnahan	Health Habits: Hygiene	1925	Elem.
Burkard, W. E., et. al.	Lyons and Carnahan	Health Habits by Practice	1926	M. El.
Burkard, W. E., et. al.	Lyons and Carnahan	Physiology and Hygiene	1926	U. El.
Emerson, C. P., & Betts, G. H.	Bobbs-Merrill Company	Living At Our Best	1926	Elem.
Jewett, Frances G.	Ginn and Company	Control of Body and Mind	1927	Elem.
Jewett, Frances G.	Ginn and Company	Good Health	1927	Elem.
Emerson, Charles P.	Bobbs-Merrill Company	Hygiene and Health	1928	Elem.
Emerson, Charles P.	Bobbs-Merrill Company	Physiology and Hygiene	1928	Elem.
Trask, John W.	D. C. Heath and Company	Essentials of Physiology	1928	Elem.
Winslow, C-E. A., & Hahn, C. H.	Charles E. Merrill Company	The New Healthy Living	1929	Elem.
Andress, James M.	Ginn and Company	Science and the Way to Health	1929	Elem.
Emerson, Charles P.	Bobbs-Merrill Company	Hygiene and Health	1930	Elem.
Emerson, C. P., & Betts, G. H.	Bobbs Merrill Company	Living At Our Best	1931	Elem.
Emerson, C. P., & Betts, G. H.	Bobbs-Merrill Company	Habits for Health	1931	Elem.
Paul, W. A., et. al.	Lyons and Carnahan	Health Habits	1931	4
Turner, Clair E.	D. C. Heath and Company	Health	1931	Elem.
Turner, Clair E.	D. C. Heath and Company	In Training for Health	1931	Elem.
Andress, James M.	Ginn and Company	Health and Success	1933	Elem.
Burkard, W. E., et. al.	Lyons and Carnahan	The Body and Health	1933	6
Wheat, Frank M.	American Book Company	Everyday Problems in Health	1933	Elem.
Brownell, C. L., et al.	Rand McNally and Company	Everyday Living	1935	Elem.
Brownell, C. L., et. al.	Rand McNally and Company	Helpful Living	1935	Elem.
Burkard, W. E., et. al.	Lyons and Carnahan	Health by Doing	1935	4
Burkard, W. E., et. al.	Lyons and Carnahan	Building for Health	1935	5
Charters, W. W., et. al.	The Macmilan Company	Keeping Healthy	1935	Elem.
Turner, Clair E.	D. C. Health and Company	The Voyage of Growing Up	1935	Elem.

Author	Publisher	Title	Date	Grade
Burkard, W. E., et. al.	Lyons and Carnahan	Building for Health	1936	5
Fowlkes, J. G., et. al.	John C. Winston Company	Healthy Living	1936	Elem.
Turner, Clair E.	D. C. Heath and Company	In Training for Health	1936	Elem.
Wood, T. D., et. al.	Thomas Nelson and Sons	Now We Are Growing	1936	Elem.
Wood, T. D., et. al.	Thomas Nelson and Sons	Keeping Fit	1936	5
Wood, T. D., et. al.	Thomas Nelson and Sons	Blazing the Trail	1936	6
Corwin, Mae G.	Harr Wagner Publishing Company	Science of Human Living	1937	Elem.
Andress, J. M., et. al.	Ginn and Company	Building Good Health	1939	6
Fowlkes, J. G., et. al.	John C. Winston Company	Keeping Well	1940	5
Fowlkes, J. E., et. al.	John C. Winston Company	Healthy Living	1940	6
Gregg, Fred M.	World Book Company	Health Studies	1940	Elem.
Burkard, W. E., et. al.	Lyons and Carnahan	Good Health is Fun	1941	4
Burkard, W. E., et. al.	Lyons and Carnahan	Health by Doing	1941	4
Burkard, W. E., et. al.	Lyons and Carnahan	Your Health & Happiness	1941	5
Burkard, W. E., et. al.	Lyons and Carnahan	Builders for Good Health	1941	6
Charters, W. W., et. al.	The Macmillan Company	Healthful Ways	1941	Elem.
Charters, W. W., et. al.	The Macmillan Company	Growing Up Healthily	1941	Elem.
Charters, W. W., et. al.	The Macmillan Company	Health Secrets	1941	Elem.
Krueger, W. W.	W. B. Saunders Company	Fundamentals of Personal Hygiene	1941	Elem.
Turner, C. E., et. al.	D. C. Heath and Company	Keeping Safe and Well	1941	Elem.
Turner, C. E., et. al.	D. C. Heath and Company	Gaining Health	1941	Elem.
Fowlkes, J. G., et. al.	John C. Winston Company	Keeping Well	1942	5
Wilson, C. C., et. al.	Bobbs-Merrill Company	Health at Home & School	1942	4
Wilson, C. C., et. al.	Bobbs-Merrill Company	Health at Work & Play	1942	5
Wilson, C. C., et. al.	Bobbs-Merrill Company	Growing Healthfully	1942	6
Brownell, C. L., & Williams, J. F.	American Book Company	Hale and Hearty	1943	5
Brownell, C. L., & Williams, J. F.	American Book Company	Active and Alert	1943	6
Phair, John T.	Ginn and Company	Good Health	1945	Elem.

Author	Publisher	Title	Date	Grade
Fowlkes, J. E., et. al.	John C. Winston Company	Healthy Growing	1948	4
Fowlkes, J. E., et. al.	John C. Winston Company	Keeping Well	1948	5
Fowlkes, J. E., et. al.	John C. Winston Company	Healthy Living	1948	6
Wilson, C. C., et. al.	Bobbs-Merrill Company	Health at Home and School	1948	4
Wilson, C. C., et. al.	Bobbs-Merrill Company	Health at Work & Play	1948	5
Rathbone, Josephine L.	Houghton Mifflin Company	Health in Your Daily Living	1952	Elem.
Jones, E., et. al.	Laidlaw Brothers	Your Health and You	1954	5
Charters, W. W., et. al.	The Macmillan Company	Growing Up Healthy	1955	Elem.

Junior High School Textbooks
1905–1955

Author	Publisher	Title	Date	Grade
Culler, Joseph A.	Lippincott Company	Second Book of Anatomy and Hygiene	1905	Jr. HS.
Conn, Herbert W.	Silver, Burdett and Company	Elementary Physiology & Hygiene	1906	Jr. HS.
Stowell, C. H.	Silver, Burdett and Company	A Healthy Body	1906	Jr. HS.
Coleman, Walter M.	The Macmillan Company	Lessons in Hygienic Physiology	1908	Jr. HS.
Davison, Alvin	American Book Company	The Human Body and Health	1908	Jr. HS.
Davison, Alvin	American Book Company	The Human Body and Health	1909	Jr. HS.
Mayberry, James W.	Southern Publishing Company	Physiology and Hygiene	1910	Jr. HS.
Millard, C. N.	The Macmillan Company	Building and Care of the Body	1910	Jr. HS.
Culler, J. A.	J. B. Lippincott Company	Anatomy, Physiology, & Hygiene	1911	Jr. HS.
Hutchinson, Woods	Houghton Mifflin Company	New Handbook of Health	1911	Jr. HS.

Author	Publisher	Title	Date	Grade
Coleman, Walter M.	The Macmillan Company	Lessons in Hygienic Physiology	1912	Jr. HS.
Coleman, W. M.	The Macmillan Company	Physiology for Beginners	1912	Jr. HS.
Hartman, Carl G.	World Book Company	The Human Body and Its Enemies	1913	Jr. HS.
O'Shea, Michael V.	The Macmillan Company	The Body in Health	1915	Jr. HS.
Conn, Herbert W.	Silver, Burdett and Company	Physiology and Health: Book 2	1916	Jr. HS.
Jewett, Frances G.	Ginn and Company	Health and Safety	1916	Jr. HS.
Wiley, Harvey W.	Rand McNally and Company	Health Reader: Physiology-Hygiene	1916	Jr. HS.
Gregg, Fred M.	By author	Hygiene as Nature Study	1917	5–8
Winslow, C.-E. A., & Hahn, M. L.	Charles E. Merrill Company	The New Healthy Living	1917	Jr. HS.
Krohn, William O.	D. Appleton and Company	Graded Lessons in Physiology and Hygiene	1919	Jr. HS.
Winslow, C-E. A.	Charles E. Merrill Company	Healthy Living: Book II	1920	Jr. HS.
Emerson, Charles P.	Bobbs-Merrill Company	Physiology and Hygiene	1921	Jr. HS.
Brown, B. M.	D. C. Heath and Company	Health in Home and Town	1922	Jr. HS.
Gregg, Fred M.	World Book Company	Hygiene by Experiment	1923	Jr. HS.
Overton, Frank	American Book Company	General Hygiene	1923	Jr. HS.
Trask, John W.	D. C. Heath and Company	Essentials of Physiology and Hygiene	1923	Jr. HS.
Davison, Alvin	American Book Company	The Human Body and Health	1924	Jr. HS.
Hartman, Carl G.	World Book Company	The Human Body and Its Enemies	1924	Jr. HS.
O'Shea, M. V., & Kellogg, J. H.	The Macmillan Company	The Body in Health	1924	Jr. HS.
Payne, E. G.	American Viewpoint Society, Inc.	We and Our Health II	1924	Jr. HS.
O'Shea, M. V., & Kellogg, J. H.	The Macmillan Company	Keeping the Body in Health	1925	Jr. HS.
O'Shea, M. V., & Kellogg, J. H.	The Macmillan Company	Building Health Habits	1925	Jr. HS.

APPENDIX

Author	Publisher	Title	Date	Grade
Payne, E. G.	American Viewpoint Society, Inc.	We and Our Health	1925	Jr. HS.
Winslow, C-E. A., & Hahn, M. L.	Charles E. Merrill Company	Healthy Living	1925	Jr. HS.
Andress, J. M., & Evans, W. A.	Ginn and Company	Health and Success	1926	Jr. HS.
Martin, Henry N.	H. Holt and Company	The Human Body	1926	Jr. HS.
Davis, Benjamin M.	Rand, McNally and Company	The Human Body and Its Case	1927	Jr. HS.
Cuzzort, Belva	D. C. Heath and Company	Health and Health Practices	1928	Jr. HS.
Newmayer, S. W., & Broome, E. C.	American Book Company	The Way to Keep Well	1928	Jr. HS.
Turner, C. E., & Collins, G. B.	D. C. Heath and Company	Community Health	1928	7–8
Winslow, C-E. A., & Hahn, M. L.	Charles E. Merrill Company	The Habits of Healthy Living	1929	Jr. HS.
Burkard, W. E., et. al.	Lyons and Carnahan	Personal and Public Health	1930	Jr. HS.
Williams, Jesse F.	Benj. H. Sanborn and Company	Health and Ideals	1930	Jr. HS.
Corwin, M. J., & Corwin, W.	Harr Wagner Publishing Company	Science of Human Living	1931	Jr. HS.
Gregg, F. M., & Rowell, H. G.	World Book Company	Health Studies	1932	Jr. HS.
Winslow, C. E. A.	Charles E. Merrill Company	The New Healthy Living	1932	Jr. HS.
Andress, J. M., & Goldburger, I. H.	Ginn and Company	The Health School on Wheels	1933	Jr. HS.
Brown, William H.	Ginn and Company	Health Through Knowledge and Habits	1933	Jr. HS.
Newmayer, S. W., & Broome, E. C.	American Book Company	Highroads to Health	1934	Jr. HS.
Winslow, C-E. A., & Hahn, M. L.	Charles E. Merrill Company	The Game of Healthy Living	1934	Jr. HS.
Brownell, C. L., et. al.	Rand McNally and Company	Happy Living	1935	Jr. HS.
Brownell, C. L., et. al.	Rand McNally and Company	Science in Living	1935	Jr. HS.

Author	Publisher	Title	Date	Grade
Charters, W. W., et. al.	The Macmillan Company	The Body's Needs	1935	Jr. HS.
Wheat, Frank M.	American Book Company	Everyday Problems in Health	1935	Jr. HS.
Brownell, C. L., et. al.	Rand McNally and Company	Progress in Living	1936	Jr. HS.
Burkard, W. E., et. al.	Lyons and Carnahan	The Body and Health	1936	Jr. HS.
Turner, C. E. & Collins, G. B.	D. C. Heath and Company	Cleanliness and Health	1936	Jr. HS.
Wood, T. D., et. al.	Thomas Nelson and Sons	How We Live	1936	7
Burkard, William E.	Lyons and Carnahan	Health and Human Welfare	1937	Jr. HS.
Wood, T. D., et. al.	Thomas Nelson and Sons	New Ways for Old	1938	Jr. HS.
Andress, James M.	Ginn and Company	Science and the Way to Health	1939	Jr. HS.
Fowlkes, J. G., et. al.	John C. Winston Company	Success Through Health	1940	7
Fowlkes, J. G., et. al.	John C. Winston Company	Making Life Healthful	1940	Jr. HS.
Wilson, C. C., et. al.	Bobbs-Merrill Company	Modern Ways to Health	1940	8
Charters, W. W., et. al.	The Macmillan Company	Habits, Healthful and Safe	1941	Jr. HS.
Charters, W. W., et. al.	The Macmillan Company	Let's Be Healthy	1941	Jr. HS.
Turner, C. E., et. al.	D. C. Heath and Company	Building Healthy Bodies	1941	Jr. HS.
Brownell, C. E., & Williams, J. F.	American Book Company	The Human Body	1942	Jr. HS.
Brownell, C. E., & Williams, J. F.	American Book Company	Living and Doing	1943	7
Brownell, C. E., & Williams, J. F.	American Book Company	Training for Living	1943	8
Burkard, W. E., et. al.	Lyons and Carnahan	Working Together for Health	1943	8
Wilson, C. C., et. al.	Bobbs-Merrill Company	Health Progress	1943	7
Wilson, C. C., et. al.	Bobbs-Merrill Company	Modern Ways to Health	1943	8
Andress, J. M., et. al.	Ginn and Company	Building Good Health	1945	Jr. HS.
Andress, J. M., et. al.	Ginn and Company	Doing Your Best for Health	1945	Jr. HS.
Brownell, Clifford L.	American Book Company	The Human Body	1946	Jr. HS.
Burkard, William E.	Lyons and Carnahan	Health for Young Americans	1946	Jr. HS.

Author	Publisher	Title	Date	Grade
Blount, Ralph E.	Allyn and Bacon	Science of Everyday Health	1948	Jr. HS.
Wilson, C. C., et. al.	Bobbs-Merrill Company	Modern Ways to Health	1948	8
Burkard, W. E., et. al.	Lyons and Carnahan	Health for Young Americans	1950	Jr. HS.
Burkard, W. E., et. al.	Lyons and Carnahan	Working Together for Health	1950	Jr. HS.
Jones, E., et. al.	Laidlaw Brothers	For Healthful Living	1954	7
Jones, E., et. al.	Laidlaw Brothers	Good Health for Better Living	1954	8
Brownell, C. L., et. al.	American Book Company	About Your Health	1955	Jr. HS.

High School Textbooks
1905–1955
(all books are simply high school)

Author	Publisher	Title	Date
Culler, Joseph A.	Lippincott Company	Third Book of Anatomy and Hygiene	1905
Pyle, W. L. (ed.)	W. B. Saunders and Company	Manual of Personal Hygiene	1905
Blaisdell, A. F.	Ginn and Company	Life and Health	1906
Hough, T., & Sedgwick, W. T.	Ginn and Company	The Human Mechanism	1906
Ritchie, John W.	World Book Company	Physiology and Hygiene	1906
Stowell, C. H.	Silver, Burdett and Company	Essentials of Health	1906
Jones, Edward G.	P. Blakiston's Son and Company	Outlines of Physiology	1908
Krohn, William O.	D. Appleton and Company	Physiology and Hygiene	1908
Overton, Frank	American Book Company	Applied Physiology	1908
Conn, H. W., & Budington, R. A.	Silver, Burdett and Company	Advanced Physiology & Hygiene	1909
Hoag, E. B.	D. C. Heath and Company	Health Studies	1909
Ritchie, J. W.	World Book Company	Physiology and Hygiene	1909
Overton, Frank	American Book Company	Applied Physiology	1910

Author	Publisher	Title	Date
Coleman, W. M.	The Macmillan Company	The Elements of Physiology	1911
Hewes, Henry F.	American Book Company	Anatomy, Physiology and Hygiene	1911
Krohn, William O.	D. Appleton and Company	Physiology and Hygiene	1912
Tolman, W. H., et. al.	American Book Company	Hygiene for the Worker	1912
Overton, Frank	American Book Company	Personal Hygiene Revised	1913
Ritchie, John W.	World Book Company	Sanitation and Physiology	1913
Ackley, Clarence E.	A. Flanagan Company	Analytical Outline of Physiology	1914
Blount, Ralph E.	Row, Peterson and Company	Physiology and Hygiene	1914
Colton, B. P., & Murbach, L.	D. C. Heath and Company	Physiology and Hygiene	1914
O'Shea, M. V., & Kellogg, J. H.	The Macmillan Company	Making the Most of Life	1915
Jewett, Frances G.	Ginn and Company	Physiology, Hygiene and Sanitation	1916
Stiles, Percy G.	W. B. Saunders Company	Human Physiology	1916
Coleman, W. M.	The Macmillan Company	Lessons in Hygienic Physiology	1917
Pyle, W. L. (ed).	W. B. Saunders and Company	Manual of Personal Hygiene	1917
Hough, T., & Sedgwick, W. T.	Ginn and Company	Elements of Hygiene and Sanitation	1918
Conn, Herbert W.	Silver, Burdett and Company	Advanced Physiology and Hygiene	1919
O'Shea, M. V., & Kellogg, J. H.	The Macmillan Company	Making the Most of Life	1919
Williams, Jesse F.	The Macmillan Company	Healthful Living	1919
Williams, Jesse F.	The Macmillan Company	Healthful Living	1920
Ritchie, John W.	World Book Company	Sanitation and Physiology	1920
Fisher, I., & Fisk, E. L.	Funk and Wagnalls Company	How to Live	1921
Blount, R. E.	Allyn and Bacon	Health: Public and Personal	1922
Goldberger, I. H., & Hallock, G. T.	Ginn and Company	Health and Physical Fitness	1923
Williams, Jesse F.	The Macmillan Company	Healthful Living	1923

Author	Publisher	Title	Date
Walters, Francis M.	D. C. Heath and Company	Physiology and Hygiene	1924
Winslow, C-E. A., & Hahn, M. L.	Charles E. Merrill Company	The Laws of Healthy Living	1924
O'Shea, M. V., & Kellogg, J. H.	The Macmillan Company	Health and Efficiency	1925
Hutchinson, Woods	Houghton-Mifflin Company	New Handbook of Health	1926
Walters, F. M.	D. C. Heath and Company	Principles of Health Control	1926
Williams, Jesse F.	The Macmillan Company	Healthful Living	1927
Winslow, C-E. A., & Hahn, M. L.	Charles E. Merrill Company	The Healthy Community	1927
Andress, J. M., et. al.	Ginn and Company	Health Essentials	1928
Jacob, A. G.	Christopher Publishing House	Personal Hygiene	1928
Meredith, F. L.	P. Blakiston's Son and Company	The Health of Youth	1928
Budington, R. A.	Silver, Burdett and Company	Physiology and Human Life	1929
Williams, Jesse F.	B. H. Sanborn and Company	Health and Service	1929
Bigelow, M. A., & Broadhurst, J.	Silver, Burdett and Company	Health for Every Day	1930
Blount, R. E.	Allyn and Bacon	Health: Public and Personal	1930
Turner, Clair E.	D. C. Heath and Company	Physiology and Health	1930
Burkard, W. E., et. al.	Lyons and Carnahan	Health and Human Welfare	1931
Walters, F. M.	D. C. Heath and Company	Our Journey of Growth	1931
Williams, Jesse F.	W. B. Saunders Company	Personal Hygiene Applied	1931
Winslow, C-E. A., & Hahn, M. L.	Charles E. Merrill Company	The New Healthy Living	1931
Gregg, F. M., & Rowell, H. G.	World Book Company	Personal Health	1932
Rathbone, J. L., et. al.	Houghton-Mifflin Company	Foundations of Health	1932
Andress, J. M., & Evans, W. A.	Ginn and Company	Health and Good Citizenship	1933
Andress, J. M., & Goldberger, I. H.	Ginn and Company	Broadcasting Health	1933

Author	Publisher	Title	Date
Williams, Jesse F.	The Macmillan Company	Healthful Living	1934
Charters, W. W., et. al.	The Macmillan Company	The Body's Needs	1935
Charters, W. W., et. al.	The Macmillan Company	Health Through Science	1935
Newmayer, S. W., & Broome, E. C.	American Book Company	Health and the Human Body	1935
Turner, C. E., & Collins, G. B.	D. C. Heath and Company	Community Health	1935
Blount, R. E.	Allyn and Bacon	Science of Everyday Health	1936
Cobb, W. F.	D. Appleton-Century Company	Health for Body and Mind	1936
Cockefair, E. A., & Cockefair, A. M.	Ginn and Company	Health and Achievement	1936
Olsson, N. W.	Globe Book Company	Guarding Our Health	1936
Rathbone, J. L., et. al.	Houghton Mifflin Company	Foundations of Health	1936
Turner, Clair E.	D. C. Heath and Company	Physiology and Health	1936
Andress, J. M., et. al.	Ginn and Company	Working Together: Health & Safety	1937
Turner, C. E., & Collins, G. B.	D. C. Heath and Company	Health	1937
Gogle, G. B.	A. S. Barnes and Company	Health for High School Girls	1938
Andress, J. M., et. al.	Ginn and Company	Working Together: Health & Safety	1939
Crisp, K. B.	J. B. Lippincott Company	Health for You	1940
Blount, R. E.	Allyn and Bacon	Science of Everyday Health	1941
Burkard, W. E., et. al.	Lyons and Carnahan	Health and Human Welfare	1941
Burnett, R. W.	Silver, Burdett and Company	To Live in Health	1941
Charters, W. W., et. al.	The Macmillan Company	Growing Up Healthily	1941
Charters, W. W., et. al.	The Macmillan Company	Health in a Power Age	1941
Charters, W. W., et. al.	The Macmillan Company	A Sound Body	1941
Crisp, K. B.	J. B. Lippencott Company	Be Healthy	1941
Turner, C. E., et. al.	D. C. Heath and Company	Working for Community Health	1941
Williams, Jesse F.	The Macmillan Company	Healthful Living	1941
Brownell, C. E., et. al.	American Book Company	Being Alive	1942
Brownell, C. E., et. al.	American Book Company	Health Problems	1942

Author	Publisher	Title	Date
Clemensen, J. W., & LaPorte, W. R.	Harcourt, Brace, and Company	Your Health and Safety	1942
Williams, J. F., & Oberteuffer, D.	McGraw-Hill Book Company	Health in the World of Work	1942
Andress, J. M., et. al.	Ginn and Company	Building Good Health	1943
Clemensen, J. W., & LaPorte, W. R.	Harcourt, Brace, and Company	Your Health and Safety	1943
Goldberger, Isidore H.	Ginn and Company	Health and Physical Fitness	1943
Burkard, W. E., et. al.	Lyons and Carnahan	Health and Human Welfare	1944
Andress, J. M., et. al.	Ginn and Company	The Healthy Home & Community	1945
Andress, J. M., et. al.	Ginn and Company	Helping the Body in Its Work	1945
Turner, C. E., & McHose, E.	C. V. Mosby Company	Effective Living	1945
Wilson, C. C., et. al.	The Bobbs-Merrill Company	Life and Health	1945
Goldberger, I. H., & Hallock, G. T.	Ginn and Company	Health and Physical Fitness	1946
Charters, W. W., et. al.	The Macmillan Company	Habits, Healthful & Safe	1947
Wheat, F. M., & Fitzpatrick, E. T.	American Book Company	Health and Body Building	1947
Wheat, F. M., & Fitzpatrick, E. T.	American Book Company	Everyday Problems in Health	1947
Bacon, L. R.	Houghton Mifflin Company	Health in Your Daily Living	1948
Wilson, Charles C.	Bobbs-Merrill Company	Life and Health	1948
McKown, H. C.	McGraw-Hill Book Company	A Boy Grows Up	1949
Williams, Jesse F.	W. B. Saunders Company	Personal Hygiene Applied	1950
Clemensen, J. W., & LaPorte, W. R.	Harcourt, Brace, and Company	Your Health and Safety	1952
Meredith, F. L., et. al.	D. C. Heath and Company	Health and Fitness	1953
Eberhardt, Charles G.	Lyons and Carnahan	Health for Better Living	1954
Williams, Jesse F.	The Macmillan Company	Healthful Living	1955

5

THE DEVELOPMENT OF A STRESS SCALE TO ASSESS BEHAVIORAL HEALTH FACTORS: THE EVERLY STRESS AND SYMPTOM INVENTORY

George S. Everly

Martin Sherman

Kenneth J. Smith

This paper reports on the development of a rapid, inexpensive, paper and pencil survey procedure for the identification of selected health-related behaviors. Specifically, the Everly Stress and Symptom Inventory (ESSI) is designed to measure three key behavioral health factors: (a) stress arousal, (b) autonomic and stress-related symptoms, and (c) behavioral coping mechanisms (divided into adaptive and maladaptive behaviors). The development of this inventory is a response to the conspicuous absence and apparent disconcern within the extant health literature for the psychometric integrity of self-report inventories that purport to assess health-related behaviors.

Our study commences with a review of the phenomenological model upon which the ESSI is based. This model includes a description of the biological and psychological components of stress arousal, the nature of coping behavior, and a measurement paradigm that outlines six potentially discrete stages of the global stress and coping phenomenon.

With the aforementioned measurement paradigm as a guide, we then proceed to describe the individual ESSI subscales. Furthermore, we report on the results of tests that have been conducted to establish the psychometric validity and reliability of each separate subscale.

Individual lifestyle and health-related behavior may be the single most important generic determinant of health status in the United States today (Public Health Service, 1979a; Green, 1981). If this conclusion is valid, as current evidence suggests, it behooves health professionals to develop a systematic method for the assessment of key health-related behaviors. The purpose of this chapter is to report on the development of a rapid, inexpensive, paper and pencil survey procedure for the identification of selected health-related behaviors.

Several lifestyles assessment surveys are already in existence within the genre of health risk appraisal instruments. For the most part, however, they represent massive surveys, which are laborious to take and impractical to score by any means other than computer. The corollary of this fact is that they are often expensive and may be difficult to interpret. Yet more importantly, a survey of the 11 most popular health risk appraisal instruments revealed a conspicuous lack of concern for psychometric validation and reliability (McMartin, 1987). It was the desire of the senior author to develop a rapid, inexpensive health-related behavior inventory that could be used for health behavior assessment as well as health education purposes that would maintain standards of psychometric integrity. Similarly, the inventory was to be practical enough for both massive health screening projects and for individual administration.

In order to achieve the aforementioned goals, it was decided that a unique approach to such assessment must be undertaken. The question was posed as to what variables might be most relevant to clinical behavioral health and medicine practices, as well as to efforts toward therapeutic health education, yet could be quickly, validly, and reliably assessed. The decision was made to draw upon epiphenomenological research in health promotion and behavioral medicine in order to isolate three key behavioral health factors: (a) stress arousal, (b) autonomic and stress-related symptoms, and (c) behavioral coping mechanisms (divided into adaptive and maladaptive behaviors). These factors were extracted from larger phenomenological models as proposed by Everly (in press); Everly and Sobelman (1987); and Lazarus and Folkman (1984). A basic phenomenological model is depicted below.

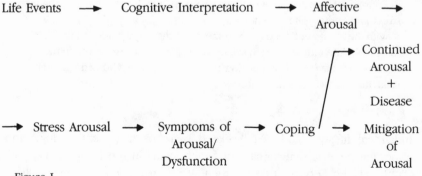

Life Events ⟶ Cognitive Interpretation ⟶ Affective Arousal

⟶ Stress Arousal ⟶ Symptoms of Arousal/ Dysfunction ⟶ Coping ⟶ Continued Arousal + Disease / Mitigation of Arousal

Figure I

This phenomenological model has been tested empirically and has been shown to possess validity through multivariate path analyses (Potocki, 1987; Dotson, Manny, & Davis, 1986). The psychometric instrument that grew out of the phenomenological model depicted in Figure I is referred to as the Everly Stress and Symptom Inventory (ESSI). The ESSI yields five subscale scores: (a) stress arousal; (b) autonomic and stress related symptoms; (c) adaptive, health promoting behaviors (A score); (d) maladaptive, health eroding behaviors (M score); (e) a "difference score" (D Score), that is, the net coping score juxtaposing maladaptive behaviors against adaptive behaviors. Let us take a closer look at the phenomenological process assessed by the ESSI.

A PHENOMENOLOGICAL MODEL

Cattell and Scheier (1961) have stated that systematic inquiry is based on some form of measurement. Furthermore, Spielberger (1975) argues that the "development of measurement procedures should be guided by a precise conceptual definition of the dimensions or variables that are to be measured" (p. 716). Unfortunately, this fundamental psychometric principle has, in many cases, been ignored in the development of instruments to measure stress arousal. As a result, a plethora of contradictory data and conclusions have appeared in the stress literature. To avoid making a similar mistake, we provide a definition that served to guide the development of the present scale.

From a biobehavioral perspective, stress may be viewed as a multifaceted physiological mechanism of mediation (i.e., a physiologic medium to bring about target-organ arousal and often a set of stress-related symptoms). The mechanism is characterized by hypermetabolic properties. This theme of hypermetabolic nature is clearly reflected in the term chosen by Nobel Laureate Walter Hess (1957) to describe one aspect of stress response: the "ergotropic response" (ergos meaning "work"). In a similar vein, Selye (1956) described stress as "the sum total of wear and tear" on the organism.

Biobehavioral researchers generally agree that stress arousal (not contingent on sympathomimetric stimulation such as caffeine, nicotine, or amphetamine consumption) is initiated by specific cognitive interpretations and resultant affective reactions on the part of the individual (Arnold, 1970; Cassell, 1974; Ellis, 1977; Everly & Rosenfeld, 1981; Gellhorn & Loofbourrow, 1963; Lazarus, 1982; Meichenbaum, 1975; Selye, 1976; Wolf, 1981a, 1981b). For example:

A concept central to many models of stress and coping is that of appraisal. This refers to the processes of evaluation and their outcomes which determine meaning, and which may or may not be conscious. There is little disagreement that it is the way in which a situation is perceived from the perspective of an individual's own history, values and expectations which is of central theoretical importance, rather than the set of characteristics ascribed to the situation on a consensual or normative basis. (Ray & Gibson, 1982, pp. 387–388)

Thus an understanding of stress can achieve conceptual clarity only through an analysis of interpretational responses (Haan, 1977), and this conclusion serves as the conceptual basis for the development of the present scale.

Examining the stress response as the generic conglomeration of physiological events that research has demonstrated it to be, three major hypothalamically derived axes emerge: the neural axis, the neuroendocrine axis, and the endocrine axis. Although these axes are multidimensional in and of themselves and in need of further understanding, some insight into their contribution to the stress response does exist.

The neural axis consists primarily of the sympathetic branch of the autonomic nervous system. Some parasympathetic action is also associated with this axis. It is thought that the effect of activating the neural axis is an immediate generalized arousal of the ergotropic system (Hess, 1957).

The neuroendocrine system appears to continue the arousal of the neural axis by way of the adrenal medullary hormones-epinephrine and norepinephrine. This response, first described by Cannon (1914), is commonly referred to as the "fight or flight" response.

Finally, the endocrine system has been shown to play an intimate role as a stress-responsive effector system. Selye (1956) provided the first clear description of the roles of the anterior pituitary, adrenal cortex, and thyroid endocrine glands in the stress response. His description of the General Adaptation Syndrome (GAS) primarily describes the functions of the glucocorticoid and mineralocorticoid hormones during stress reactivity.

In sum, the hypermetabolic stress response represents activation of neural, neuroendocrine, and endocrine mechanisms now known to be capable of classic signs and symptoms of psychosomatic-psychophysiological disorders. The physiological response is a function of an individual's cognitive and affective reactions to environmental conditions (stressors) in which the individual finds oneself, not the actual conditions themselves. We should also note that as the physiological stress response initiates, numerous and diverse end-organ signs and symptoms emerge. These signs and symptoms may include a wide range of psychological, behavioral, or physiological manifestations (see Everly & Rosenfeld, 1981). Finally, when faced with excessive arousal or discomfort, organisms attempt to cope so as to avoid target-organ disease.

COPING

Coping is defined as efforts, both action-oriented and intrapsychic, to manage (that is master, tolerate, reduce, minimize) environmental and internal demands, and conflicts among them, which tax or exceed a person's resources. Coping can occur prior to a stressful confrontation, in which case it is called anticipatory coping, as well as in reaction to a present or past confrontation with harm. (Cohen & Lazarus, 1979, p. 219)

Coping behavior can be dichotomized as either "adaptive" or "maladaptive" to further clarify the concept. Adaptive coping is defined as any coping behavior that can be used to manage demands and reduce stress/anxiety while simultaneously fostering/promoting personal health. Examples include relaxation techniques, exercise, etc. Maladaptive coping represents any coping behavior that can be used to manage demands and reduce acute stress/anxiety but which is simultaneously self-debilitating in that such behavior will create other demands and prolonged stress/anxiety. Examples might include smoking, eating to cope with stress, drug abuse, etc. It is important to note that both adaptive and maladaptive coping behaviors are usually effective in reducing *acute* demands and stress and anxiety. Yet maladaptive coping behaviors will tend to generate longterm demands and stress/anxiety on their own, whereas adaptive coping behaviors tend to foster health and reduce demands and stress/anxiety in the long run. It is insufficient to limit measurement to adaptive or maladaptive behavior, however. Data exist that strongly infer consideration of adaptive behavior vis-a-vis maladaptive behavior as the ultimate determinant of health status. Research by Bradburn (1969), Lowenthal and Chiriboga (1973), and Gersten et. al. (1974) present data supporting consideration of the "balance" between health-enhancing and health-debilitating behaviors.

A Measurement Paradigm

To understand the ESSI fully, it seems important to consider the paradigm from a systems perspective. Based on the previous discussion we can argue that the global phenomenon consists of: (a) the environment (stressors), (b) the cognitive-affective reactions to the environment, (c) the stress response itself (the physiological axes), (d) the psychosomatic signs and symptoms of the stress response, (e) coping mechanisms (see Everly & Sobelman, 1987), and (f) disease. Thus, six potentially discrete stages actually exist in the global response paradigm.

Not only do these stages help clarify what the phenomenon actually is, but they also serve as a model for understanding the measurement dilemma that surrounds stress and related concepts, as well as providing a basis for developing a measurement tool. In effect, by using the conceptual formulation above, it becomes clear that important health factors might be measured from any of these six points, that is: (a) quantification of environmental stressors; (b) the assessment of the cognitive-affective domain; (c) the actual assessment of one or more physiological axes, that is, the stress response itself; (d) the end-organ signs and symptoms of stress arousal; (e) coping behaviors; and (f) measures of disease.

The ESSI assesses the most clinically relevant and pragmatic of these domains: (a) the cognitive-affective domain, (b) the autonomic symptom domain, and (c) coping mechanisms.

The self-report of the individual's cognitive-affective domain provides an indirect yet superior form of stress assessment. In this process we are able to gain insight into a person's own perceptual sphere concerning self, environment, and self-environment interaction (the key determinant of the elicitation of the stress response as reviewed earlier). Although self-report can be fraught with biases and defense mechanisms, Derogatis (1977) states that "the self-report mode of psychological measurement contains much to recommend it" (p. 2). This is especially true vis-a-vis the stress response. Speed of data accumulation and interpretation is enhanced. Cost is low even in large scale settings (e.g., training environments, classroom formats, large clinics, and even occupational-vocational assessment). Frequent retesting is easily accommodated (e.g., to test the effectiveness of a stress management course or therapy). The above reasons motivated the development of the present scale utilizing a self-report of the cognitive-affective reactions that initiate the stress response.

The actual measurement of the stress response would necessarily entail assessment of the three major physiological axes. Such activities are often invasive (therefore requiring medical supervision), expensive, (up to several hundred dollars per assessment per person), time consuming (taking 1–2 days for interpretation), subject to diurnal fluctuation and sampling bias, and generally impractical.

Measurement of the psychosomatic end-organ symptoms will be achieved through the use of a self-report autonomic and symptom-related checklist. Coping will be assessed via self-report of adaptive and maladaptive coping strategies.

THE STRESS AROUSAL SCALE

As noted earlier the stress arousal phenomenon will be assessed indirectly through the use of 20 items selected as indicators of cognitive-affective arousal.

Research on the arousal scale was initiated (by Everly) in 1976. Item pools were generated that best appeared to represent theoretically compatible cognitive-affective precipitants of the stress response. Although it cannot be indisputably proven that various cognitive-affective conditions cause activation of the stress response, it is now generally accepted that these conditions are highly correlated with stress arousal. Under this premise the development of a paper and pencil self-report scale that identified theoretically compatible cognitive-affective variable conditions highly correlated with the presence of the stress response was undertaken.

The scale asks respondents how often they have recently ("within the last few weeks") experienced each of the 20 cognitive-affective conditions. Respondents are asked to select from four options—almost always, often, sometimes, or seldom or never—for each of the 20 items (see Table I). For example:

How often have you found yourself satisfied?   1. Seldom or Never
                                                 2. Sometimes
                                                 3. Often
                                                 4. Almost Always

The scale contains several safeguards aimed at avoiding some of the potential problems of self-report scales. The 20 primary items contain 4 "reversed" items to compensate for response patterning. In addition, an earlier version of the ESSI was correlated with the Marlowe-Crowne Social Desirability Scale (Crowne & Marlowe, 1964) to assess the former's potential to be influenced by respondents' social desirability needs, thus invalidating

TABLE 1
Selected Arousal Scale Items

How often have you found yourself disappointed?
How often have you found yourself frustrated?
How often have you found yourself happy?
How often have you found yourself hassled?
How often have you found yourself upset?
How often have you found yourself secure?
How often have you found yourself annoyed?

the scale's responses. The correlation for 36 respondents was −.21 ($p = .10$). The nonsignificance of this relationship suggests a low vulnerability to the influence of social desirability under normal response conditions. Finally, the scale was field tested on over 100 professional educators. A consensus indicated that the items could be understood and responded to by individuals possessing a ninth grade education.

Reliability

The scale has shown its metric reliability. Reliability is defined as the tendency of a psychometric instrument to yield consistent responses. The test-retest reliability of the scale was .88 and .95 over a one-week interval in independent studies of 42 and 22 asymptomatic individuals, respectively.

The internal consistency of the scale was assessed using the alpha coefficient. In a sample of 1026 adults (age $\bar{x} = 25.2$, $SD = 10.9$) drawn from the states of Colorado, Maryland, Delaware, and Kentucky, the coefficient alpha was found to be .947. See Table II.

TABLE 2
Correlations Between Items and Corrected Total Score
(Total Score minus Item)

Item	Item-Totals Corrected	Alpha
1	.629	.945
2	.601	.945
3	.645	.944
4	.636	.945
5	.652	.944
6	.732	.943
7	.695	.944
8	.646	.944
9	.735	.943
10	.736	.943
11	.653	.944
12	.567	.946
13	.674	.944
14	.585	.946
15	.688	.944
16	.720	.943
17	.703	.944
18	.749	.943
19	.718	.943
20	.628	.945

In a subsample of 882 adults equally divided by gender, the standard error of measure was found to be 2.51 for all subjects, 2.47 for males, and 2.53 for females.

Validity

The validity of the arousal scale was assessed through the use of concurrent discriminant validity, construct validity, and path analysis.

The ability of a scale to concurrently differentiate subjects who possess the trait (arousal) from those who do not is called concurrent discriminant validity. Prodromidis (1986) found that the arousal scale was able to correctly identify over 96% of a group of 41 stress-related disease patients. She further found that the scale could correctly identify 90% of a group of 40 anxiety patients. Finally, she found that the scale could correctly identify over 85% of carefully screened asymptomatic subjects ($n = 41$). Potocki (1987) found that the scale could correctly identify 85% of a population self-referred to an addictions treatment facility ($n = 77$). A subsequent study found that the scale could correctly identify over 81% of a morbidly obese female population ($n = 70$).

To assess the construct validity of the arousal scale, the scale was correlated with existing measures of relevance to the construct of stress arousal. Prodromidis (1986) found that the scale correlated with the STAI (Trait) with a magnitude of .82 for 40 anxiety patients, .52 for 41 stress-related disease patients, and .71 for 41 asymptomatic subjects. All correlations are meaningful and in the predicted directions. Potocki (1987) found the scale to correlate with a magnitude of .78 with the premorbid pessimism scale on the Millon Clinical Multiaxial Inventory for a sample of 79 subjects from an addictions screening facility. She also found that the scale correlated with a magnitude of .377 with self-reports of drug abuse.

An investigation of 70 morbidly obese females found the scale to correlate .73 with the Beck Depression Inventory, .689 with the Depression scale of the SCL-90, .68 with the Anxiety scale of the Millon, .64 with the Dysthymia scale on the same inventory, .70 with the Anxiety scale of the SCL-90, and .64 with the Hostility scale of the SCL-90. All of these correlations are meaningful and in the predicted direction.

Finally, the arousal scale was phenomenologically assessed via path analysis methods to assess its role in a multivariate phenomenological model of stress and illness. The arousal scale was found to assess a statistically meaningful and theoretical congruent aspect of the phenomenological model described earlier in the paper (Dotson et al., 1986; Potocki, 1987).

Repeated studies with the arousal scale have found differences to occur according to gender. It is therefore recommended that in order to maximize discriminant power a cutting line of 48 be established for males and a cutting line of 50 be established for females. Scores above these lines can generally be thought of as having an 82% or greater chance of making a true positive diagnosis of pathogenic stress arousal. In a normally distributed population of males that aggregates symptomatic with asymptomatic individuals, it may be expected that approximately 27% of the population will score above 48 (n = 441): in a normally distributed population of females that aggregates symptomatic with asymptomatic individuals, it may be expected that approximately 29% of the population will exceed a score of 50 (n = 441). The aforementioned samples were drawn from the states of Maryland, Delaware, Kentucky, and Colorado and represent what data suggest may be the normative base rate prevalent of stress arousal as measured by this scale. Mean values for carefully screened asymptomatic groups have shown to be 35.68 (SD = 8.21), whereas such values for carefully diagnosed stress-related disease patients have been found to be 52.34 (SD = 6.04), and 54.40 (SD = 9.94) for a sample of carefully diagnosed anxiety disorder patients.

THE AUTONOMIC SYMPTOM SCALE

It was believed that a brief inventory of symptoms of autonomic nervous system dysfunction would be a valuable addition to the assessment tool under construction. Therefore, 38 items were generated to tap this domain.

The Autonomic Conditions Checklist (ACC) is a list of bodily conditions that individuals sometimes experience. Respondents are asked to indicate using the following response options how often they recently ("in the last few weeks") have been experiencing each condition; 0 = not at all, 1 = less than once a week, 2 = once or twice a week, 3 = more than twice a week (see Table III). A person's total score is calculated by simply summing the scores selected for each individual question.

Reliability

The test-retest reliability of the symptom inventory was found to be .89 for 93 college students using a 1-week interval ($\bar{x}$ score = 23.9, SD = 15.45).

Validity

The validity of the symptom inventory was demonstrated in the path analyses performed by Dotson et al. (1986) and Potocki (1987).

TABLE 3
Selected Autonomic Conditions Checklist Items

Listed below are a number of bodily conditions that people sometimes experience. Please use the numbers provided to describe how often you have *recently* (in the last few weeks) been experiencing each condition. Place that number in the space to the left of each condition listed below. This is *not* a test—there are no right or wrong answers. Simply respond to this checklist as quickly and honestly as you can.

0—Not at all
1—Less than once a week
2—Once or twice a week
3—More than twice a week

_____ Upset stomach
_____ Neckaches
_____ Change in appetite
_____ Muscle tightness
_____ Heart pounding
_____ Nervousness

Further construct validation was provided by correlating the symptom inventory with other indices. In a sample of 70 morbidly obese females, the scale was found to have the following relationships: .63 with the Anxiety scale on the Millon Clinical Multiaxial Inventory, and .60 with the Dysthymia scale on that inventory; .56 with the Anxiety scale of the SCL-90, .46 with the depression scale of the SCL-90, and .75 with the Global Symptom Index of the SCL-90. Potocki (1987) found the symptom inventory to correlate with the Millon Premorbid Pessimism subscale, .56; and with the Life Events Inventory, .37—all among a group of 79 individuals self-referred to an addictions screening facility.

THE ESSI COPING SCALE

The coping scale on the ESSI is designed to be a survey of adaptive and maladaptive coping behaviors. It contains 20 questions: 10 related to adaptive coping behaviors, and 10 related to maladaptive coping behaviors. The questions ask respondents whether they engage in specific coping techniques in their daily lives. Respondents generate three scores. The *A* score indicates the number of adaptive coping behaviors respondents engage in by summing the number of *yes* responses on the odd-numbered questions. Yes responses to the even numbered questions yields an *M* score, which reflects the maladaptive coping behaviors exhibited. The third score is termed the *D* score and represents the residual score after subtracting the *M* score from the *A* score. The *D* score provides an indication of the overall health-enhancing behavior practiced by individual respondents.

The following sections on validity and reliability primarily address the *D* score. This is the only score on the scale that an attempt was made to use in a scaler fashion. The rationale for utilizing the *D* score was, again, a reflection of its role as a "balance" between health-enhancing and health-eroding behaviors. We should note that the *A* and *M* scores retain their utility as health behavior checklists despite the psychometric emphasis on the *D* score.

Reliability

The test-retest reliability of the *D* score over a one-week interval for 34 graduate students and 13 undergraduate students was .74 ($p<.001$) and .75 ($p<.05$), respectively. Over a two week interval, the test-retest reliability of the *D* score was .75 ($p<.01$) for 12 graduate students in another investigation. These coefficients are within acceptable limits.

Validity

Theoretic validity for the coping scale was determined upon the basis of "expert" consensus. That is, item generation for the scale was based upon a review of the literature within the domains of health-enhancing and

TABLE 4
Selected Coping Scale Items

Do you have a supportive family of group or friends close by that you would rely on for help if you needed it?

Do you smoke one-half or more packs of cigarettes in an average day?

Do you exercise at least 3 times a week for twenty minutes or longer each time?

Do you eat more to help you cope with high levels of pressure, stress, or anxiety?

During an average week, do you take any form of medication or chemical substance (including alcohol) to help you sleep?

Do you practice time management techniques in your daily life? (Time management techniques include delegation, prioritization, and scheduling of your work and home tasks.)

---

health-eroding life-style behaviors (see Grawunder & Steinman, 1980; Public Health Service, 1979b; Girdano & Everly, 1986). Items were reviewed by a group of experts representing the fields of medicine, psychology, and health education to assure that the items adequately represented the desired behavioral domains.

Construct validity for the scale was assessed by seeking divergent correlational validity. The D score was correlated with the Taylor Manifest Anxiety Scale generating a $-.40$ coefficient ($p<.001$) for 295 undergraduate students. The D score correlated with the trait version of the State Trait Anxiety Inventory at a $-.34$ level ($p<.001$) for the same 295 undergraduates. These correlations are in the predicted direction and are supportive of the D score as an index of health-enhancing behavior. Similarly, the D score was correlated with the stress arousal scale at the $-.35$ level ($p<.001$) for 96 undergraduate students. This relationship is also in the predicted direction.

Concurrent criterion validity was tested on the basis of the contrasted groups procedure. As illustrated in Table V, the D score was able to differentiate groups of psychophysiologic patients from nonclinical subjects. In essence, the D score can discriminate between clinical and nonclinical

TABLE 5
t-tests for clinical vs. nonclinical groups on the D scale

GROUPS	MEANS	SD	t-values	p
137 undergraduates	2.67	2.43	3.76	$p<.001$
17 clinicals (group A)	.176	2.59		
20 light industrial workers	3.75	2.76	5.16	$p<.001$
17 clinicals (group A)	.176	2.59		
295 undergraduates	2.28	2.62	3.25	$p<.001$
17 clinicals (group A)	.176	2.59		
137 undergraduates	2.67	2.43	2.12	$p<.05$
10 clinicals (group B)	1.00	2.40		
20 light industrial workers	3.75	2.76	2.81	$p<.01$
10 clinicals (group B)	1.00	2.40		
17 clinicals (group A)	.176	2.59	.787	$p<.05$ (n.s.)
10 clinicals (group B)	1.00	2.40		

groups although failing to discriminate between two different clinical groups. These results are supportive of the *D* score's ability to identify health-enhancing behavior patterns.

SUMMARY

The present paper has reported on the development of a psychometrically based, health-related behavior inventory. The rationale for the development of this inventory grew out of a conspicuous absence and apparent disconcern within the extant health-related literature for the psychometric integrity of self-report inventories that purport to assess health-related behaviors. This point is graphically demonstrated by several factors: (a) McMartin's (1987) review of health-related instruments, which totally ignored critical psychometric criteria in her evaluative process; (b) the dearth of substantiated psychometric properties within instruments that purport to assess the health behavior domain; and (c) the minimal amount of psychometric training provided in schools of public health, health education, and medicine.

The Everly Stress and Symptom Inventory was born of the senior author's desire to integrate selected principles of psychometric development with the assessment of the health behavior domain. More specifically, the ESSI purports to assess stress arousal, autonomic nervous system symptomotology, and three domains of coping (health-promoting coping behavior, health-eroding coping behavior, and the net difference in coping behavior). The present paper has demonstrated that the ESSI does indeed satisfy basic psychometric requirements in the assessment of the aforementioned health-related behaviors and symptoms. In doing so, it may be suggested that the ESSI serves as a contribution to the endeavors of health education and health-related assessment. For the fundamental epistemological issue that undergirds the conduct of inquiry is nothing less than the reliability and validity of the data upon which we make health-related decisions, be those decisions diagnostic, educational, or treatment oriented. The ESSI as reported herein will be further researched so as to refine its epistemological integrity; nevertheless, in its present form data argue for its current utility.

REFERENCES

Arnold, M. (Ed.). (1970). *Feelings and Emotions.* New York: Academic Press.
Bradburn, N. (1969). *The Structure of Well-being.* Chicago: Aldine.
Cannon, W. (1914). The emergency function of the adrenal medulla in pain and in the major emotions. *Journal of Physiology. 33,* 356–372.

Cassell, J. (1974). Psychosocial processes and stress: Theoretical formulation. In *The Behavioral Sciences and Prevention Medicine* (pp.   ) Washington, DC: U.S. Public Health Service.

Cattell, R. B., & Scheier, I. H. (1961). *The Meaning and Measurement of Neuroticism and Anxiety.* New York: Ronald Press.

Cohen, F., & Lazarus, R. (1979). Coping with the stresses of illnesses. In G. Stone, F. Cohen, & N. Adler *Health Psychology* (pp. 217–254). San Francisco: Jossey-Bass.

Crowne, D., & Marlowe, D. (1964). *The Approval Motive.* New York: Wiley.

Derogatis, L. (1977). *SCL-90(R) Manual-I.* Baltimore: Author.

Dotson, C., Manny, P., & Davis, P. (1986). *A Study of Occupational Stress Among Poultry and Red Meat Inspectors.* Langley Park, MD: The Institute of Human Performance.

Ellis, A. (Ed). (1977). *Handbook of Rational Emotive Therapy.* New York: Springer.

Everly, G. (in press). *A Clinical Guide to the Treatment of the Human Stress Response.* New York: Plenum.

Everly, G., & Rosenfeld, R. (1981). *The Nature and Treatment of the Stress Response.* New York: Plenum.

Everly & Sobelman. (1987). *The Assessment of the Human Stress Response.* New York: AMS Press.

Gellhorn, E., & Loofbourrow, G. (1963). *Emotions and Emotional Disorders.* New York: Harper & Row.

Gersten, J., et. al. (1974). "Child behavior and life events". In B. S. Dohrenwend & B. P. Dohrenwend (Eds.) *Stressful Life Events* (pp. 159–170). New York: Wiley.

Girdano, D., & Everly, G. (1986). *Controlling Stress and Tension. Vol. II.* Englewood Cliffs, NJ: Prentice-Hall.

Grawunder, R., & Steinmann, M. (1980). *Life and Health.* New York: Random House.

Green, L. (1981, July). *Emerging federal perspectives on health promotion.* Health Promotions Monographs, Whole No. 1.

Haan, N. (1977). *Coping and Defending.* New York: Academic Press.

Henry, J., & Stephens, P. (1977). *Stress, Health, and the Social Environment.* New York: Springer.

Hess, W. (1957). *The Functional Organization of the Diencephalon.* New York: Grune and Stratton.

Lazarus, R. (1966). *Psychological Stress and the Coping Process.* New York: McGraw-Hill.

Lazarus, R. (1982). *Thoughts on the relations between emotions and cognition.* American psychologist, *37,* 1019–1024.

Lazarus, R., & Folkman, S. (1984). *Stress Appraisal and Coping.* New York: Springer.

Lowenthal, M., & Chiriboga, D. (1973). Social stress and adaptation". In C. Eisdorfer & M. Lawton (Eds.), *The Psychology of Adult Development and Aging* (pp. 281–310). Washington, DC: American Psychological Association.

McMartin, E. J. (1987). Shopping for Health Risk Appraisals, Part II. *Health Action Managers, 1,* 4–9.

Meichenbaum, D. (1975). A self-instructional approach to stress management. In C. Spielberger & I. Sarason (Eds.), *Stress and Anxiety, Vol. I* (pp.   ). New York: Wiley.

Potocki, E. (1987). *Premorbid pessimism as a modifier between life events, stress, and illness.* Master's thesis, Loyola College.

Prodromidis, M. (1986). *The Use of a Cutting Line to Discriminate Symptomatic from Asymptomatic Subject Groups.* Master's thesis: Loyola College.

Public Health Service. (1979a). *Healthy People: The Surgeon General's Report on Health Promotion and Disease Prevention.* Washington, DC: U.S. Government Printing Office.

Public Health Service. (1979b). *Healthy People: The Surgeon General's Report on Health Promotion and Disease Prevention—Background Papers.* Washington, DC: U.S. Government Printing Office.

Ray, C. Lindop, Jr., & Gibson, S. (1982). The concept of coping. *Psychological Medicine, 12,* 385–395.

Selye, H. (1956). *The Stress of Life.* New York: McGraw-Hill.

Selye, H. (1976). *Stress in Health and Disease.* Boston: Butterworth.

Spielberger, C. D. (1975). The measurement of state and trait anxiety. In L. Levi (Ed.), *Emotions-Their Parameters and Measurements* (pp.   ). New York: Raven Press.

Wolf, S. (1981a). *The psychosocial forces and neural mechanisms in illness and disease.* Paper presented at the Samuel Novy Lectureship in Psychological Medicine, Johns Hopkins University, Baltimore.

Wolf, S. (1981b). The role of the brain in bodily disease. In H. Weiner, M. Hofer, & A. Stunkard (eds.), *Brain, Behavior, and Bodily Disease.* New York: Raven Press.

6

PROFESSIONAL PREPARATION IN WORKSITE HEALTH PROMOTION

Randall R. Cottrell

Lorraine G. Davis

Jane M. Gutting

The purpose of this study was to obtain information regarding the current status of health promotion professional preparation programs in America. A survey was mailed to a random sample of colleges and universities with professional preparation programs in health education. Results of this survey indicate that over half of all colleges and universities preparing professional health educators currently have specific programs available in worksite health promotion. These programs can be found in all geographic regions of the country and typically are jointly administered by health education and physical education departments. The programs have a variety of titles, but emphasis on fitness is common. Exercise prescription, first aid, nutrition/diet management, stress management, and weight control are the most important and most frequently required content courses. Evaluation procedures, statistics and research methods are the most frequently required process-type courses. Private health clubs and large businesses are seen by colleges and universities as the most likely sites of employment for their graduates. Hospitals, public employee's groups, and colleges and universities were also seen as possible sites of employment.

The number of worksite health promotion programs in the United States has skyrocketed in the past ten years. Recent estimates suggest that as many as 50,000 organizations may currently be involved in health promotion activities (Howe, 1983; Jacobs, 1983). This represents a dramatic increase from the estimated 75 companies providing health and fitness programs for their employees in 1973 (Hoffman & Hobson, 1984). A few of the highly visible corporate health promotion programs are those of Metropolitan Life, Xerox, Control Data, Kimberly Clark, Campbell Soup, Tenneco, and Pepsico. Nearly 30% of the Fortune 500 companies have health promotion programs in place for their employees with an additional 5% ready to initiate programs (Forouzesh, 1985).

The proliferation of worksite health promotion programs has occurred for many reasons, but essentially these programs have potential benefits for employers, employees, and health promotion professionals. Employers look to health promotion programs to reduce employee health care costs, absenteeism and voluntary turnover; to increase productivity and employee morale; to aid in the recruitment of new personnel; and to generally improve the corporate image (O'Donnell & Ainsworth, 1984).

While the objectives for employees in health promotion programs include an enhanced overall quality of life and improved health status, the immediate benefits should not be overlooked. Participants receive low direct-cost health promotion services, conveniently located at the worksite (Everly & Feldman, 1985). Health promotion providers benefit by gaining access to an isolated population (Chen & Jones, 1982). Since American adults spend slightly over one-third of their working hours at their worksite, employees are not available to take advantage of many community health or school health promotion strategies. In addition, compliance of employees participating in health promotion programs at the worksite may be high; colleagues can offer mutual support; and health behavior change becomes an integral component of one's work life.

As worksite health promotion programs continue to grow in both number and complexity, the need for qualified health professionals will become critical (Golaszewski, Tomik, Pyle, & Pfieffer, 1983). Chenoweth (1983) has stated; "The quest to recruit the qualified professional has met with less than favorable results, possibly due to a market saturated with individuals lacking competence in the health sciences. Currently, the demand exceeds the supply for qualified health management personnel." It has been predicted that between 1985 and 1995 the majority of major industries in the United States will employ health educators to implement wellness programs (Toohey & Shirreffs, 1980). If this prediction becomes reality, colleges and universities involved in professional preparation of health educators will need to address both philosophical and curricular concerns. An evaluation of whether or not existing curricula prepare students to develop and deliver worksite health promotion programs will have to be made.

The literature has discussed the content of a singular health promotion course (Chen & Jones, 1982), the competencies desired of health personnel from a corporate viewpoint (Golaszewski et al., 1983; Seehafer, Black, Hiner, & Melby, 1985), and the curricular guidelines for a professional preparation program for health promotion specialists (Chenoweth, 1983). No definitive data are available regarding the current status of programs preparing professionals for worksite health promotion or what typical programs include.

The purpose of this study was to obtain data concerning the preparation of professionals in health promotion in terms of programs available, coursework required, coursework deemed important, and potential job opportunities for worksite health promotion graduates. This information is useful for individuals with established programs for comparative purposes; as baseline data for those initiating programs; and to contribute to the documentation and development of worksite health promotion professional preparation (HPPP) programs.

METHODS

A survey was developed to collect data regarding the status of worksite HPPP programs. Questions were asked to ascertain whether or not a specific independent program to train students for health/fitness management positions existed. If such programs did exist, questions were asked to determine the level of preparation (BS, MS, PhD), the official name of the program, and the department that housed the program. Next, a list of 25 possible content areas appropriate for health promotion professionals were presented. Each professional content area was selected for inclusion in the questionnaire if it was identified in the literature or if it was part of any known program. Courses in each content area were identified as "required," "elective," or "not offered" by survey respondents. Additionally, each course content area was ranked on a 5-point Likert scale from "very important" to "not important." Finally, respondents were requested to rate a list of various worksite settings as to the "likelihood of employment" for graduates of HPPP programs.

A random sample of 200 institutions offering undergraduate and/or graduate professional preparation in Health Education was selected from the 1985 AAHE Directory of Institutions (Moore, 1984). Surveys were addressed to "Director Health/Fitness Management Program" and mailed to each of the selected institutions. Respondents were requested to complete the survey whether or not they had a professional preparation program.

RESULTS

Of the 200 surveys mailed, 101 usable surveys were returned for a response rate of 51%. Fifty-four (53.5%) of the responding institutions indicated they currently had a specific independent program, other than school health, community health, or physical education, designed to place students in health/fitness management positions. An additional 19 (40%) respondents anticipate offering a separate HPPP program option within the next two years. Overall, 72% of the respondents reported either currently having programs or planning programs within the next two years.

No significant regional differences in the number of institutions offering professional preparation programs were noted. Comparisons by region as shown in Table I indicate that the percentage of questionnaires returned, the percentage of programs offered, and the percentage of questionnaires mailed were very similar. Over 50% of respondents from each region of the United States reported having specific independent programs in existence. The central region was the only section of the country reporting over 60% of colleges and universities with specific HPPP programs.

Questions were asked to determine the academic level at which professional preparation in health/fitness management is taking place. Of the 54 respondents with programs, 41 (76%) offered programs at the bachelors level, 14 (44%) offered programs at the masters level, and 4 (7%) offered programs at the PhD level. Only two programs offered special certificate programs in HPPP.

HPPP programs were housed in various college and university departments. Twenty-five (46%) of the HPPP programs were jointly housed in health and physical education departments. Seventeen programs (32%) were

TABLE 1
Percentage of Sample Sent, Percentage of Returned, and Percentage with Programs by Region

Region	Sample Sent		Returned		With Programs	
	N	%	N	%	N	%
South	66	33	27	29	16	31
East	45	23	18	20	10	19
Midwest	40	20	19	21	10	19
Central	20	10	11	11	7	13
Southwest	16	8	10	9	5	10
Northwest	13	6	7	7	4	8

located solely in physical education departments and 8 programs (15%) were located solely in health education departments. Business departments and other non-health/physical education departments housed 4 programs (7%).

Very little standardization exists as to the title of programs designed to place students in worksite settings. Of the 54 institutions responding, 23 (43%) had fitness or physical education titles with no mention of health. Thirteen programs (24%) used titles reflecting both health and fitness. Health or wellness was used with no mention of fitness or physical education by 9 programs (17%). Nine additional programs (17%) made no mention of either health or fitness in their titles. Community Service, Sports Medicine, Lifelong Sport Management, and Biodynamics are examples of such titles.

Respondents to the survey who had HPPP programs in place were asked to examine a list of 25 possible course offerings and identify which courses were "required," which were available as "electives," and which were "not offered." Results of this process can be seen in Table 2. Of the most frequently required courses, 6 were health foundation/knowledge courses. Of those 6 content courses, 2 dealt with first aid, 2 were exercise related, and 2 focused on diet and weight control. The remaining 4 of the most frequently required courses were related to program planning and evaluation. Least often required, but most frequently offered as "electives" were courses related to aging, drug use, human behavior, and counseling. Courses in occupational health and safety were neither required nor offered by the majority of respondents.

All respondents were asked to rank each of the 25 potential course offerings on a Likert scale from very important (1) to not important (5). Using numerical values, means were calculated for each course offering. Table 3 presents the mean rankings from "most important" to "least important." When comparing the required course rankings with the perceived importance of courses very little difference in the 5 top ranked courses appear. The bottom 3 courses also remained essentially the same. Some shifts in ranking did occur. Both statistics and research methods, which were ranked comparatively high in the required course table, were ranked much lower on the perceived importance table. Other course offerings that had a drop of at least five positions from the required course table to the perceived importance table include: first aid, drug use/abuse, and business management. Courses in motivating human behavior and public relations were not frequently required but were considered important. Courses in tobacco use were also seen as fairly important, but were not frequently identified as required.

The final component of the questionnaire asked respondents to rank potential work settings as to the likelihood of employment for HPPP

TABLE 2
Health Promotion Courses Required, Elective, and Not Offered

Course	Req.	Elec.	Not Offered	Missing
1. EXERCISE PRESCRIPTION	43	5	1	5
2. FIRST AID	40	12	1	1
3. EVALUATION PROCEDURES	38	7	5	4
4. NUT/DIET MANAGEMENT	37	15	0	2
5. CPR	35	17	1	1
6. STATISTICS	34	6	9	5
7. RESEARCH METHODS	28	3	14	9
8. FITNESS MANAGEMENT	27	8	11	8
9. WEIGHT CONTROL	26	13	7	8
10. PROGRAM PLANNING	26	13	9	6
11. STRESS MANAGEMENT	26	14	9	5
12. BUDGETING/FINANCIAL MGMT	25	16	8	5
13. ORGANIZATIONAL MANAGEMENT	22	17	11	4
14. INTERPERSONAL COMMUNICATION	19	15	15	5
15. BUSINESS MANAGEMENT	18	19	8	9
16. DRUG USE/ABUSE	16	27	6	5
17. MARKETING	16	23	7	8
18. MOTIVATING HUMAN BEHAVIOR	16	22	10	6
19. ALCOHOL USE/ABUSE	15	24	9	6
20. TOBACCO USE	14	21	13	6
21. COUNSELING METHODS	13	24	13	4
22. PUBLIC RELATIONS	11	21	12	10
23. SAFETY	11	18	20	5
24. AGING/GERONTOLOGY	6	29	13	6
25. OCCUPATIONAL HEALTH	3	16	26	9

graduates. Each of six potential worksite settings were ranked on a 5-point Likert scale ranging from "definitely a site of employment" (5) to "very unlikely to be a site of employment" (1). Results of the mean score calculations for each employment site can be seen in Table 4. Private health clubs and large businesses were seen as the most likely sites of employment for HPPP graduates. All but small businesses had mean scores between 3 and 4, indicating they are possible to likely sites of employment.

DISCUSSION

From the results of this survey, over 50% of institutions preparing health educators currently have specialized programs (other than school or community health) to prepare students for careers in worksite health

TABLE 3
Perceived Importance of Health Promotion Course

Course	Mean Rating*
1. NUT/DIET MANAGEMENT	1.34
2. EXERCISE PRESCRIPTION	1.38
3. FITNESS MANAGEMENT	1.51
4. CPR	1.57
5. WEIGHT CONTROL	1.58
6. EVALUATION PROCEDURES	1.60
7. STRESS MANAGEMENT	1.64
8. MOTIVATING HUMAN BEHAVIOR	1.71
9. FIRST AID	1.72
10. INTERPERSONAL COMMUNICATION	1.76
11. PROGRAM PLANNING	1.82
12. BUDGETING/FINANCIAL MGMT	2.06
13. TOBACCO USE	2.07
14. PUBLIC RELATIONS	2.10
15. MARKETING	2.11
16. STATISTICS	2.12
17. ORGANIZATIONAL MANAGEMENT	2.13
18. ALCOHOL USE/ABUSE	2.15
19. COUNSELING METHODS	2.15
20. RESEARCH METHODS	2.17
21. DRUG USE/ABUSE	2.23
22. BUSINESS MANAGEMENT	2.27
23. AGING/GERONTOLOGY	2.40
24. SAFETY	2.42
25. OCCUPATIONAL HEALTH	2.91

*Scale values range from 1 to 5; 1 indicates very important.

TABLE 4
Rating of Worksite Health Promotion Employment Potential

Job Site	Mean Rating*
PRIVATE HEALTH CLUBS	3.990
LARGE BUSINESS	3.780
HOSPITALS	3.337
PUBLIC EMPLOYEE GROUPS	3.103
COLLEGES/UNIVERSITIES	3.010
SMALL BUSINESS	2.808

N = ALL 101 RESPONDENTS TO SURVEY
*Scale values range from 1 to 5; 5 indicates employment very likely.

promotion. Ethically, health educators must be certain they do not prepare more students for jobs in worksite health promotion than the market can bear. Although more and more worksites are initiating health promotion programs, how many are seeking qualified health educators to fill these positions? HPPP programs preparing students for health promotion careers must take the responsibility to help students get placed. Making direct contact with companies, hospitals, and health spas in the immediate area is one way this can be accomplished. In addition, articles need to be written in business journals to inform corporate decision makers that specialists in health promotion are available.

The level of preparation needed for students to best serve in the worksite setting is another concern that must be addressed. From this survey the majority of students are being trained at the bachelor's level. This is probably sufficient for positions emphasizing direct program delivery to clients; for other positions requiring detailed program planning, implementation strategies, and evaluation procedures, the skills provided in a masters degree program may be more appropriate. Institutions need to decide if one level of preparation is appropriate for them or if preparation needs to be provided at both the bachelor's and master's level. Again, corporate decision makers need to be educated as to the difference between the two degree programs and what can be expected of their respective graduates.

Most programs preparing students for careers in worksite health promotion are operated jointly from health education and physical education departments, or from combined health/physical education departments. This is a natural combination since most worksite health promotion programs include both exercise/fitness and traditional health education topics such as nutrition, weight control, smoking cessation, and stress management. Despite the fact that programs have a joint health education/physical education emphasis, most program titles reflect fitness. Perhaps this is because fitness is the most visible aspect of many corporate programs. Another possible explanation stems from the fact that, traditionally, fitness programs have been the first health promotion efforts for many companies. Even the professional organization, the Association for Fitness in Business, emphasizes fitness in its title, instead of a broader health promotion or wellness focus. Certainly fitness is an integral component of health promotion efforts, but problems may occur by placing too much focus on one element. To many people outside the health education and physical education fields, the term fitness means exercise; not the broader concept of total individual fitness that includes other health related behaviors. Employers hiring someone to conduct broad-range health promotion programs may perceive someone trained as a "fitness specialist" to be only capable of conducting exercise programs. The use of more comprehensive terms in the title of worksite professional preparation programs such as health promotion or health/fitness management would serve to reduce such problems.

In general, courses that provide process skills such as organizational management, marketing, public relations, and budgeting/financial management, fell in the middle range of importance and frequency required. Courses providing specialized content knowledge were identified as being more important and more frequently required. Substance abuse courses (tobacco, alcohol, drugs) were noted exceptions to this trend. They ranked in the bottom half of courses for both frequency required and perceived importance. Given the number of worksite Employee Assistance Programs that address these issues and their relative cost effectiveness when compared to other topical areas, these findings were somewhat unexpected. One possible explanation for the relative low ranking of the substance abuse topics is that such programs when offered at the worksite are often contracted from consultants or private organizations; therefore, the health promotion professional may not have as much need for in-depth skill training in these areas. In addition, substance abuse issues are not as "safe" to confront as other topic areas discussed at the worksite, and probably the complexity of the issue makes professional preparation difficult. Ethical considerations, particularly confidentiality, must be addressed in professional preparation courses focusing on substance abuse. At the very least students preparing for worksite health promotion careers need to be provided with an understanding of substance abuse problems and what resources are available to help with these issues.

Survey results showed that safety and occupational health courses were not required, not offered, and not even deemed important in professional preparation programs. Initially, these ratings would seem unusual, but when considered in conjunction with the ratings of potential employment settings, logical explanations surface. In large businesses and private health clubs responsibility for safety and occupational health would be assumed by professionals in those areas, and rightly so. In some of the other employment situations, particularly in small businesses, the health promotion specialist would be likely to have responsibilities in the safety area. Given the dicotomous nature of employment situations, the amount of coursework desirable for every graduate remains ambiguous.

The ideal coursework requirements necessary in aging/gerontology, are more obvious but nonetheless were deemed unimportant. Given that health promotion professionals work with people throughout the life span, an understanding of the aging process is imperative. Another factor to support the inclusion of aging/gerontology courses in professional preparation programs is the increasing population of persons in the older age categories. Perhaps people have an inaccurate perception regarding the content of aging/gerontology coursework and think that the age groups studied are limited to retirement and beyond.

Employment trends for health promotion professionals could logically change from those indicated in the current survey results. Large businesses and private health clubs will likely remain as employment possibilities. The potential for small business as worksite health promotion clients exists. Employment in a consultant role or as a member of a private corporation planning and delivering health promotion may be more feasible than the traditional direct employment avenue for worksites with smaller numbers of personnel. Creative innovative techniques for providing health promotion service could be considered and even taught as part of professional preparation programs.

If HPPP programs are developed, curricular planning needs to include an evaluation component as a segment of the process. This study was an investigation of existing programs. Results were reported with regard to programs available, curricular content, and potential job opportunities for graduates.

The next logical step would be to survey employers of health/fitness management programs to determine their priorities and expectations in the professional preparation of health/fitness management specialists. Hopefully, existing professional preparation programs are philosophically compatible and content specific to the goals of current health/fitness worksite programs. Finally, graduates of HPPP programs need to be studied with regard to opinions about their professional preparation. As currently employed health/fitness program managers, was their education adequate? As newly developed HPPP programs move forward, it is imperative they are under constant evaluation and revision. These programs are providing the foundation for a new profession. University and college faculty must be responsible in assessing the compatibility of their professional preparation goals to the goals of the worksite. Are health/fitness management curriculum writers and employees of health/fitness specialists marching to the beat of the same drum?

REFERENCES

Chen, M. S., & Jones, R. M. (1982). Preparing health educators for the workplace: A university-health insurance company alliance. *Health Values: Achieving High Level Wellness, 6,* 9–12.

Chenoweth, D. (1983). Health education in the private sector: Preparing tomorrow's health management personnel. *Health Education, 14,* 28–34.

Everly, G. S., & Feldman, R. H. L. (1985). Occupational Health Promotion. New York: John Wiley & Sons.

Forouzesh, M., & Ratzker, L. E. (1985). Health promotion and wellness programs: An insight into the Fortune 500. *Health Education, 15,* 18–21.

Golaszewski, T., Tomik, W., Pyle, R., & Pfieffer, G. (1983). Competency identification, evaluation and improvement for corporate health program fitness specialists: Health education variables. *Health Education, 14,* 28–34.

Hoffman, J. J., & Hobson, C. J. (1984). Physical fitness and employee effectiveness. *Personnel Administrator, 29,* 101–113.

Howe, C. (1983). Establishing employee recreation programs. *Journal of Physical Education, Recreation and Dance, 54,* 34–52.

Jacobs, B. A. (1983). Sound minds, bodies . . . and savings. *Industry Week, 216,* 67–68.

Moore, L. M. (1984). AAHE directory of institutions offering specialization in undergraduate and graduate professional preparation programs in health education, 1985 edition. *Health Education, 15,* 80–88.

O'Donnell, M. P., & Ainsworth, T. (1984). Health Promotion in the Workplace. New York: John Wiley & Sons.

Seehafer, R., Black, D. R., Hiner, G. C., & Melby, C. L. (1985). Health promotion competencies: Implications from a survey of program administrators. *The Eta Sigma Gamman, 17,* 2–6.

Toohey, J. U., & Shirreffs, J. H. (1980). Future trends in health education. *Health Education, 11,* 15–17.

7

WORKSITE HEALTH PROMOTION PROGRAMS IN MIDSIZE NEW JERSEY FIRMS: SURVEY FINDINGS

Roberta B. Hollander

Joseph J. Lengermann

A study was carried out to examine the nature of worksite health promotion programs in midsize New Jersey manufacturing firms. In addition to looking at which companies had health promotion programs, this study explored the number and types of activities offered; employee eligibility and participation; organizational support, that is, who pays and on whose time employees participate in activities; what types of personnel are employed in health promotion programs; and whether firms carry out planning activities, including needs assessments, evaluations, and cost analyses. These issues were examined in relation to the variables of type of industry and organization size. The sample totaled 174 firms with a response rate of 50.6%.

Study findings indicate that 35% of the respondents have worksite health promotion programs and 44% of these plan to expand their program offerings. For those firms without programs, 13% have plans to initiate them. Size of organization was found to be significantly and directly related to the existence of programs, the mean number of health promotion activities, and whether companies planned to expand or initiate programs. In general, type of industry also had a bearing on the extensiveness of worksite programs. Other study findings, including those related to the use of planning and evaluation techniques, suggest as well that organization size and, to a lesser degree, type of industry are variables of interest in examining health promotion programs in the workplace.

Recent surveys of worksite health promotion programs document the extent to which such programs are being adopted by a growing number of companies in the United States. Much of the research on programs in work settings, however, has been limited to larger firms, such as the Fortune 500, and has not examined closely how programs differ depending on size, the type of industry, and other characteristics of the parent organizations. Accordingly, the purpose of this article is to contribute to the effort to describe and assess modes of growth of health promotion programs in various types of work organizations. In order to extend our understanding of worksite health promotion programs in midsize and smaller companies, the results of a survey of health promotion programs in a sample of New Jersey manufacturing firms are reported. Findings from the present study are compared with results from other research on worksite programs, particularly with respect to the variables of size of organization and industry type. Study findings are also presented concerning whether organizations in the sample have programs; the nature and extent of activities offered within programs; the extent of employee eligibility and participation in the programs; and whether these work organizations carry out planning activities, including needs assessments, evaluations, and cost analyses.

RESEARCH ON ORGANIZATIONAL DIFFERENCES IN WORKSITE HEALTH PROMOTION

Worksite health promotion efforts in Fortune 500 companies have been the focus of two recent surveys, one reported by Hollander and Lengermann (1988) and an earlier study by Forouzesh and Ratzker (1984/1985). Forouzesh and Ratzker found that 29.3% of responding Fortune 500 companies offered worksite health promotion programs to their employees, compared with the two-thirds of respondents in the Hollander and Lengermann study that had programs of this order. Forouzesh and Ratzker also reported that, for their respondents, the specific types of companies that were most likely to have programs were petroleum and oil-producing companies, followed by metal manufacturers.

In addition to examining the extent to which companies had health promotion programs and the nature of these programs, the study by Hollander and Lengermann (1988) explored these characteristics in light of the organizational variables of size (number of employees), Fortune 500 rank, and type of industry (high versus low technology). The results indicated that, in general, the larger, higher ranked and high technology companies were more likely to have programs; offer more activities in programs; have plans for program expansion; use a model of the employer and the employee sharing costs of activities and time off to participate in activities; make greater use of health professionals; and utilize needs assessment, evaluation, and cost analysis techniques.

Size has emerged as a variable of interest in other studies of worksite health promotion as well. For example, Fielding and Breslow's work regarding California companies (1983), the research by Davis, Rosenberg, Iverson, Vernon, and Bauer. (1984) in Colorado, a study by Danielson and Danielson (1980) in Ontario, and the work by Dean, Reid, and Gzowski (1984) also in Ontario have all found that health promotion programs are more likely to be established in larger work organizations.

Herzlinger and Calkins (1986) and others (Shain, Suurvali, & Boutilier, 1986) have examined the impact of industry type on worksite health promotion efforts. Herzlinger and Calkins (1986) found that program offerings differ according to industry type. For example, oil, steel, finance, and insurance companies are more likely to offer smoking related programs, whereas mining, chemical, oil, transportation, communications, entertainment, and utility industries tend to offer alcohol and drug programs. Other health promotion activities were also found to vary by industry type. Similarly, in a study of industrial manufacturing plants in South Carolina, Chovil, Alexander, Gibson, and Altekruse (1983) found that the occupational health services provided varied according to type of industry. The level of health services offered (basic, secondary, or tertiary) in most cases was also affected by the number of employees.

METHODS

For the present study, questionnaires were sent to 383 manufacturing plants in the state of New Jersey during the spring of 1987. Eighty-three of these plants were the same as those selected by random sample and included in a previous study of organizational characteristics and industrial innovation in New Jersey manufacturing firms (Hull and Hage, 1980). It is anticipated that the set of data on organizational characteristics and industrial innovation from the previous study and the present data set on worksite health promotion programs will be examined in conjunction with one another in a future article. The remaining 300 manufacturing plants to which our questionnaires were sent were selected, for purposes of analysis, in order to achieve a more substantial sample size on a range of size categories.

The *New Jersey Directory of Manufacturers* (1984) was used to draw a stratified random sample of manufacturing firms. This annual publication lists by geographic area and product line all manufacturing firms within the state that employ more than five persons. A table of random numbers was used to generate the sample with selection into three strata of plant size based on the number of employees in the plant: 200–499 employees, 500–1000 employees, and more than 1000 employees. The ratio of plants selected for the sample to estimated number of plants in the total population for these three groups was: 100 to 1550, 100 to 475, and 100 to 800, respectively.

The instrument used in this study was similar to that previously used by the authors in their survey of Fortune 500 companies (Hollander & Lengermann, 1988). In addition to eliciting information about the nature and extent of health promotion activities in these firms, the questionnaire addressed characteristics of the firms, and whether they conducted planning and evaluation activities with respect to their health promotion programs.

Questionnaires were sent directly to each of the plant managers, with a request that they be completed either by someone in this position or by the most appropriate person (e.g., the health or medical officer). The cover letter and instructions requested that respondents answer the questionnaire in terms of the local plant, if possible, or else in terms of the entire company, and to indicate the unit for which they were answering. Although respondents were asked to list specific health promotion activities, most questions were asked in reference to the program as a whole. No formal definitions of health promotion or wellness programs were provided. Rather, respondents answered on the basis of their own perceptions whether such a program exists in their plant or company. The likelihood of misunderstanding was lessened by providing a list at the beginning of the questionnaire of the 10 health promotion activities most frequently cited in the literature. Shain et al. (1986), and Hollander and Lengermann (1988) have used this approach in other research on worksite programs. Two follow-up mailings were carried out in an effort to maximize the response rate.

With respect to the category breakdowns for the major independent variables of size and type of industry, size was operationally defined in terms of the number of employees. Respondents were asked how many employees they had in their local plant and how many in their entire company. Each measure of size is used separately in the following analysis. The size categories for each of these measures were determined by dividing up the respondent companies around substantively meaningful breaking points. The three category breakdown for plant size is: less than 200 (42%), 200–499 (39%), and 500–5,000 (18%). (Due to rounding, percentages do not always add up to 100.) Note that because many plants had decreased in size since the compilation of the directory and because many respondents focused specifically on the local plant unit to which the questionnaire had been sent, a considerable proportion (42%) of the plant units reported on had somewhat fewer than 200 employees. For size of company (for which fewer repondents provided information) the three categories are: less than 500 (30%), 500–2999 (35%), and 3,000–99,998 (35%). Because it is reported in the organizational literature that the impact of size diminishes as the size of organizations increases, it was expected that size would be even more important in the present study than in the survey of the Fortune 500 companies (Blau, 1970).

The type of industry for respondent companies was taken from the standard industrial classification (SIC) codes provided for each plant/company in the *New Jersey Directory of Manufacturers* (1984). These four-digit codes, which represent the principle product lines for companies, initially are analyzed at the two-digit level for descriptive purposes. Industries are then categorized along a low-technology/high-technology (lo-tech/hi-tech) dimension on the basis of four-digit code industry level research and development (R & D) expenditure. R & D expenditure is often taken as a proxy measure of technological intensity (Freeman, 1982; Shanklin & Ryans, 1984). Although there is some debate about the most meaningful R & D level for distinguishing between low and high technological intensity (Davis, 1982), we will rely here principally on a below average versus above average breakdown. Thus, plants and companies that are primarily in industries in the lower fiftieth percentile in terms of their coefficient of technological intensity (R & D cents per dollar of shipments) are categorized here as lo-tech (68%), and those in the upper fiftieth percentile as hi-tech (32%). If one prefers to follow the recommendation of Lester Davis (1982) that the most relevant criterion for high technological intensity is not whether an industry is above the average in R & D but whether, in statistical terms, it is "significantly above the average," it is appropriate to note here that all but nine of the 55 respondent firms classified here as hi-tech and all but one of the 24 hi-tech firms that have worksite health promotion programs, are in fact in industries that are in the "significantly above average" group.

Frequency distributions, cross tabulations, and analysis of variance techniques are used in the analysis of the data. The reported levels of significance in the tables are based on chi square for cross tabulation percentages and on the F statistic from the analysis of variance for relationships for which means are reported. Checks for interaction effects were carried out by cross tabulation and three-way analysis of variance. However, results are reported primarily in terms of the more direct bivariate analyses.

RESULTS

The response rate for the survey was 50.6%, based on 174 useable responses received from a list of 344 plants. Thirty-nine companies from the original list of 383 were judged to fall out of the sample because of information that the company had gone out of business or had moved with no forwarding address. Of the 174 respondents 54% answered in terms of the local plant and 46% answered in terms of the company as a whole.

Extensiveness of Programs and Activities

We first examine how many plants/companies in our New Jersey sample have a worksite health promotion program and what activities are offered. For the first question, respondents were requested to simply circle a yes or no response. For the latter question, they could check any or all of eleven health promotion activities and could write in others not on the list. In total, 22 activities were coded. Respondents were also asked if their plant or company had plans to start up or expand programs and to list specific activities related to such plans.

As suggested in Table 1, there is only a low to moderate amount of worksite health promotion activity in these New Jersey manufacturing plants. Only 35% of the responding New Jersey companies reported that they have some kind of worksite health promotion program. Not surprisingly, given the differential availability of resources, this is considerably lower than that previously found in the study of Fortune 500 companies (Hollander & Lengermann, 1988). It is also lower than the rate reported for a national sample of companies (Windom, McGinnis, & Fielding, 1987). The mean number of activities included in the New Jersey programs was somewhat lower than that found in Fortune 500 companies two years ago, 6.4 versus 7.9. Additionally, the New Jersey firms are considerably lower than the Fortune 500 group in the percentage of companies without programs that have plans to initiate programs (13% compared to 33%), as well as in the percentage of companies with programs that have plans to expand their programs (44% compared to 61%). Contrary to expectations, those respondents who completed the questionnaire on the basis of their local plant site report a higher rate of having programs than those who did so on the basis of their entire company (42% compared to 26%). The explanation for this seems to lie in the fact that those responding on the basis of their local plant site also are more likely to come from the larger plants and companies.

It is highly unlikely that these lower figures are the result of a reversal in the popularity of these programs during the past two years or to less interest in worksite health promotion within New Jersey. As Table 1 clearly shows, the size of the plant or company makes a tremendous difference in whether or not organizations have programs and the number of activities offered. New Jersey plants and companies in the largest of our size categories in fact show somewhat higher levels of having programs, having more activities in

TABLE 1
Extent of Worksite Health Promotion Programs in New Jersey
(N = 174) and Fortune 500 Firms (N = 249)

	% (n) of Companies with Programs	Mean # of Activities in (n) Programs	% (n) with Plans to Begin if Do Not Have Programs	% (n) with Plans to Expand if Already Have Programs
Total New Jersey	35 (61)	6.4 (61)	13 (15)	44 (25)
Total Fortune 500	66 (164)	7.9 (164)	33 (26)	61 (92)
Plant Size-NJ				
001–199	24 (13)**	4.5 (13)***	5 (2)***	33 (4)
200–499	44 (23)**	6.0 (28)***	21 (6)***	44 (10)
500–5000	70 (16)**	9.0 (16)***	71 (5)***	57 (8)
Company Size—NJ				
001–499	20 (12)**	4.3 (12)	11 (5)	58 (7)
500–2999	36 (15)**	6.8 (15)	19 (5)	36 (5)
3000–99998	59 (13)**	6.7 (13)	11 (1)	46 (5)
Type of Industry—NJ				
Lo-Tech	22 (34)**	6.0 (34)	10 (8)	41 (14)
Hi-Tech	44 (24)**	6.9 (24)	23 (7)	50 (10)

* $P<.05$
** $P<.01$
*** $P<.001$

programs, and planning to begin or expand programs than do the Fortune 500 companies. The relationships between each of these two dimensions of size and having worksite health promotion programs are consistently maintained when controlling for the other dimension. The relationships also hold when controlling for whether respondents completed the questionnaire in terms of their local plants or their entire companies. It would seem then that: (a) size appears to be a very critical factor in the extensiveness of worksite health promotion programs and that (b) once size is controlled for, worksite health promotion is even more common now than indicated in studies of two years ago. Type of industry, in terms of lo-tech or hi-tech, also seems to have a bearing on the extensiveness of worksite health promotion, although not as much as the variable of size. Hi-tech companies, for the most part, seem to have a somewhat greater involvement in worksite health promotion programs.

We can also construct a picture of which specific program activities are most prevalent and whether or not their prevalence is related to size and industry factors. Table 2 lists, in rank order, the ten most common worksite activities and the percentage of companies that offer these activities. The much lower prevalence of most of these activities in the New Jersey sample relative to the Fortune 500 companies is immediately obvious. So, too, is the strong impact of size within the New Jersey sample and, to a much lesser degree, that of type of industry. As for differences between the New Jersey and Fortune 500 samples regarding which activities are most commonly offered, only a few activities show markedly different rankings. Accident prevention ranks as the most common offering in the New Jersey sample for all size and industry groupings but only as the fourth most common activity in the Fortune 500 companies (tied with smoking cessation and fitness/exercise). Fitness/exercise is much more common in the Fortune 500 companies and in the larger New Jersey companies (rank 4) than in the New Jersey sample as a whole (rank 9) or in the smaller New Jersey companies (rank 8).

Characteristics of Organizational Support for Programs

A variety of characteristics of the New Jersey worksite health promotion programs were examined that bear on the question of the amount and nature of organizational resources devoted to them. First of all, we asked about the origin of the program—whose idea it was to start the worksite health promotion program. Of the 57 companies who responded to this question, 28% attributed responsibility to the parent company, 32% to company managment, 16% to on-site health professionals, and 25% to employee groups or unions (but in combination with management). The size of the plant or company was not significantly related to which group was responsible for initiating the program. Hi-tech companies were slightly more likely ($p < .07$) than their lo-tech counterparts to attribute the ideas to parent company management (33% compared to 24%) and to employee/union groups (28% compared to 22%).

Second, respondents were asked who pays for worksite health promotions programs (the organization, the employees, or a combination of both) and what percentages of the costs were borne by employer and employees respectively. Results are reported in Table 3. Overall, 63% of the respondents reported that the employer paid for all the costs, 7% reported that employees paid for all the costs, and 30% reported that costs were paid by some combination of employers and employees. The mean percentage of worksite health promotion costs reported as paid by employers was 86%. These

TABLE 2
Prevalence of Specific Activities in Worksite Health Promotion Programs in New Jersey (N = 61) and Fortune 500 (N = 164) Firms

	NJ-Total (n = 61) Rank—%	Fort .500 (n = 164) Rank—%	NJ-Small Companies (n = 13) Rank—%	NJ-Large Companies (n = 16) Rank—%	NJ-Lo-Tech Companies (n = 34) Rank—%	NJ-Hi-Tech Companies (n = 24) Rank—%
Accident Prevention	1–98	4–75	1–92	1–100	1–100	1–98
Hypertension, BP Control	2–70	1–83	3–53	2–88	2–68	2–71
Health Risk Assessment	3–65	2–78	2–77	9–44	5–44	3–67
Alcohol, Drug Assistance	4–49	3–76	4–46	4–63	3–53	5–46
Smoking Cessation	5–46	4–75	5–39	3–81	4–47	5–46
Health Education	6–43	—	5–39	8–50	5–44	7–42
Cancer Screening, Control	7–33	7–65	9–8	7–56	10–24	4–50
Weight Control, Nutrition	8–32	7–65	7–23	4–63	7–29	8–38
Fitness, Exercise	9–30	4–75	8–15	4–63	7–29	9–33
Stress Management	10–29	9–61	10–7	9–44	7–29	10–29

TABLE 3
Who Pays and Whose Time Used in Worksite Health Promotion Programs in New Jersey (N = 61) and Fortune 500 (N = 164) Firms

	Whose Time Used in Program			Who Pays for Program		
	% (n) Company Time Only	% (n) Employee Time Only	% (n) Combined Time	% (n) Company Pays All	% (n) Combined Payment	Mean % Paid by Companies (n)
Total New Jersey	41 (25)	16 (10)	43 (26)	63 (38)	30 (18)	86.0 (45)
Total Fortune 500	20 (31)	31 (48)	50 (78)	53 (81)	43 (66)	84.2 (133)
Plant Size—NJ						
001–199	54 (7)	23 (3)	23 (3)	85 (11)*	8 (1)*	86.8 (13)
200–499	48 (10)	5 (1)	48 (10)	68 (15)*	27 (6)*	91.5 (15)
500–5000	27 (4)	27 (4)	47 (7)	38 (6)*	50 (8)*	75.1 (13)
Company Size—NJ						
001–999	55 (6)	9 (1)	36 (4)	67 (8)*	17 (2)*	76.2 (9)
1000–2999	15 (2)	31 (4)	54 (7)	53 (8)*	48 (7)*	91.5 (11)
3000–99998	39 (5)	23 (3)	39 (5)	77 (10)*	23 (3)*	95.2 (11)
Type of Industry—NJ						
Lo-Tech	41 (14)	12 (4)	47 (16)	68 (23)	29 (10)	93.7 (23)
Hi-Tech	41 (9)	23 (5)	36 (8)	58 (14)	29 (7)	77.8 (22)

* $P < .05$
** $P < .01$
*** $P < .001$

figures are comparable to those reported in a previous study of Fortune 500 companies, though with the New Jersey firms reporting slightly higher levels of company payment. Size of plant is related to who pays, with the smaller plants paying a larger proportion of program costs. This is most clearly the case for those responding on the basis of their local plant, with 85% of the smallest size category, 68% of the midsize category, and only 38% of the largest category reporting that the company paid all costs, while 8%, 27%, and 50% of these same categories reported that a combination of employer and employee payment is used (p <.05). Size of company, however, as well as type of technology do not seem to be related to the pattern of payment for worksite health promotion costs in this sample.

A related question to who pays for worksite health promotion activities is whose time is used to participate in them. The data are presented in Table 3. Overall, 41% of the respondents report that activities are carried out entirely on company time, 16% on employees' own time, and 43% on some combination of employer and employee time. The comparable figures for Fortune 500 companies are 20%, 31%, and 50%. Plant size, and to some extent company size have some impact, with the larger plants and companies being less likely to offer health promotion activities entirely on company time but more on a combination of company and employee time. Type of industry has some impact in that hi-tech companies are inclined to have activities occur more on employees' own time and less on combined time than are the lo-tech companies. The lower levels of company support by the larger and hi-tech New Jersey companies for activities being offered on company time (as well as the generally lower levels of such support among the New Jersey companies relative to the Fortune 500 companies) is very likely related to the previously discussed pattern of the type of activities offered (greater predominance of activities such as exercise rather than accident prevention) and by the higher number of activities offered.

A final aspect of the extent and nature of organizational resources being devoted to worksite health promotion programs in New Jersey companies is a consideration of the kinds of personnel utilized in the implementation of the programs. As we see in Table 4, the New Jersey firms are somewhat less likely than Fortune 500 firms to utilize health professionals. Plant size and company size (but not technological intensity) are related consistently and postively to the greater use of health professionals, whether we look at the use of a specific practitioner group (health educators, nurses, physicians) or a combination of such groups. Fitness experts also are seen to be utilized more extensively by the larger plants and companies as well as by the more hi-tech companies. This is consistent with their greater emphasis on exercise and fitness in their worksite health promotion programs.

TABLE 4
Types of Personnel Employed in Worksite Health Promotion Programs in New Jersey (N = 61) and Fortune 500 (N = 164) Firms

	% (n) with Personnel Officers	% (n) with Fitness Experts	% (n) with Health Educators	% (n) with Nurses	% (n) with Physicians	% (n) with at least 1 Type Health Professionals	% (n) with at least 2 Types Health Professionals	% (n) with at least 3 Types Health Professionals
Total New Jersey	46 (26)	14 (8)	28 (16)	65 (37)	46 (26)	81 (47)	50 (29)	16 (9)
Total Fortune 500	39 (60)	—	39 (60)	74 (115)	60 (93)	83 (136)	59 (97)	23 (37)
Plant Size—NJ								
001–199	69 (9)	8 (1)*	31 (4)	31 (4)*	46 (6)	69 (9)	39 (5)	8 (1)
200–499	59 (13)	5 (1)*	27 (6)	64 (14)*	46 (10)	77 (17)	55 (12)	9 (2)
500–5000	31 (5)	31 (5)*	25 (4)	94 (15)*	50 (8)	94 (16)	59 (10)	29 (5)
Company Size—NJ								
001–999	42 (5)	8 (1)	33 (4)	33 (4)***	17 (2)***	58 (7)	33 (4)	0 (0)
1000–2,999	47 (7)	20 (3)	33 (5)	53 (8)***	47 (7)***	80 (12)	60 (9)	13 (2)
3000–99998	42 (5)	17 (2)	33 (4)	92 (11)***	67 (8)***	93 (12)	69 (9)	23 (3)
Type of Industry—NJ								
Lo-Tech	46 (15)	12 (4)	30 (10)	70 (23)	52 (17)	82 (28)	56 (19)	18 (6)
Hi-Tech	46 (11)	17 (4)	25 (6)	58 (14)	38 (8)	79 (19)	42 (10)	13 (3)

* $P<.05$
** $P<.01$
*** $P<.001$

Eligibility and Participation

Given the preceding information about the extensiveness of, and organizational support for, worksite health promotion programs in New Jersey firms, there remains the question of how effective such programs are in reaching workers. Eligibility refers to how many and what types of employees have the opportunity to participate; as such, it represents another aspect of the extensiveness of worksite health promotion programs in companies. Respondents were asked to provide an estimate of the percentage of employees eligible to participate in worksite health promotion programs. Because of concerns about questionnaire length, a limitation is that this question was asked in reference to entire programs rather than about specific health promotion activities. The relatively high levels reported in Table 5

TABLE 5
Eligibility and Participation Rates in Worksite Health Promotion Programs in New Jersey ($N = 61$) and Fortune 500 ($N = 164$) Firms

	Mean % Employees Eligible in (n) Programs	Mean % Participation by Eligible Males in (n) Programs	Mean % Participation in Activity Most Popular for Females in (n) Programs	Mean % Participation in Activity Most Popular for Males in (n) Programs
Total New Jersey	96.4 (49)	51.2 (44)	55 (30)	59 (26)
Total Fortune 500	89.4 (131)	40.1 (99)	—	—
Plant Size—NJ				
001–199	98 (10)	63 (9)**	66 (7)*	72 (7)
200–499	94 (18)	63 (16)**	69 (9)*	69 (7)
500–5000	98 (14)	28 (15)**	33 (11)*	40 (9)
Company Size—NJ				
001–999	91 (11)	61 (9)	62 (6)	70 (5)
1000–2,999	98 (13)	48 (11)	54 (7)	53 (6)
3000–99998	98 (12)	44 (10)	45 (8)	39 (6)
Type of Industry—NJ				
Lo-Tech	90 (30)	54 (26)	71 (14)**	71 (14)*
Hi-Tech	94 (19)	47 (18)	42 (16)**	45 (12)*

* $P < .05$
** $P < .01$
*** $P < .001$

must be understood in these terms. The mean percentage of employees reported eligible for at least one kind of worksite health promotion activity in New Jersey firms is 96.4%. This is somewhat higher than, though comparable to, the 89.4% of employees reported eligible in the study on Fortune 500 companies. Plant size, company size, and type of technology do not have much bearing on this issue, at least when the question does not address eligibility for specific activities.

Given such high levels of eligibility, what percentage of workers take advantage of this opportunity and actually participate in worksite health promotion programs? If programs are to result in the desired health and cost outcomes, it is critical that programs not just be put in place but that employees participate in them. Thus, the rate of participation can be seen as an intermediate indicator of program effectiveness. Again, the questionnaire requested that respondents estimate the percentage of workers who participate in the program as a whole, rather than in specific activities. This approach, in conjunction with the usual potential biases in self-reported data, increases our expectation that the results will be somewhat inflated relative to actual participation. Nevertheless they provide a rough and meaningful barometer on this issue. The fact that the reported levels of participation in Table 5 are so much lower than the reported levels of eligibility gives us some confidence in the data, as well as some concern that worksite health promotion programs are not reaching nearly as many employees as they could. The reported mean participation rate for males (rates for females are almost identical at the general level) in New Jersey firms is 51.2%. This is slightly higher than the 40.1% reported in our study of Fortune 500 firms. Contrary to the Fortune 500 data for participation rates, which show a weak but consistent tendency to vary positively with size and technological intensity, the New Jersey data show a strong tendency for size and technological intensity to relate negatively to participation. This finding is consistent with results from previous studies of midsize firms, and particularly with the Canadian study by Dean et al. (1984). The questionnaire also asked respondents to name the activities in which their employees participated the most and the percentage of employees who participated in these activities. Differences between males and females in their preferences for various worksite health promotion activities appeared. Therefore, Table 5 reports participation rates separately for the two gender groups. The impact of plant size, company size, and technological intensity again appears to be strong and to relate negatively to participation levels for both males and females. Some of these differences in participation rates can be understood in terms of the difficulty in larger organizations to motivate employees to participate in organizational programs of any kind, but some of these differences are also likely to be due to the previously discussed factor of differences in the kinds of worksite health promotion programs emphasized according to size and technology. Attaining widespread participation in such programs as exercise, weight reduction, and hypertension may be more problematic than getting employees to participate in accident prevention, particularly because accident prevention programs are often mandatory.

Planning, Needs Assessment, Evaluation, and Cost Analyses

As with the study on Fortune 500 firms, New Jersey companies were also asked whether they had carried out formal planning procedures, including needs assessments, evaluations, and cost analyses in their worksite health promotion programs. The use of these planning and evaluation techniques can be interpreted as reflecting the level of organizational commitment to worksite health promotion programs as well as a harbinger of their eventual success and stabilty. The application of these techniques to worksite health promotion programs in Fortune 500 firms was found to be quite low (Hollander & Lengermann, 1988.) As expected, Table 6 shows that their use in the New Jersey firms is even lower, with 67% of the companies reporting that they use none of the three specific techniques and only 41% reporting that formal planning procedures had been applied in the development of their programs. Only 24% reported using needs assessment, 19% reported using evaluation, and 16% reported using cost analysis. Comparable figures for Fortune 500 firms were 41%, 35%, and 16%, respectively. Although size and rank were only weakly related to the use of these techniques among Fortune 500 firms, both plant size and company size appear to be clearly and positively related to their use in the sample of New Jersey firms.

CONCLUSION

This study of midsize New Jersey manufacturing firms supports the belief that worksite health promotion programs have spread beyond the elite Fortune 500 and other large-scale companies to a wide variety of work organizations. The findings also suggest that programs exist at the plant level almost as commonly as on the general company level.

Study results clearly point to the importance of taking into account various organizational characteristics in the description and assessment of worksite health promotion programs. As evident in this study, worksite programs differ in the number and types of activities offered, their levels of com-

TABLE 6
Use of Needs Assessment, Evaluation, and Cost Analysis Techniques in Worksite Health Promotion Programs in New Jersey ($N = 61$) and Fortune 500 ($N = 164$) Firms

	% (n) Using General Planning	% (n) Using Needs Assess.	% (n) Using Evaluation	% (n) Using Cost Analysis	% (n) Using None at all	% (n) Using One Tech.	% (n) Using Two Tech.	% (n) Using Three Tech.
Total New Jersey	41 (23)	24 (14)	19 (11)	16 (9)	67 (39)	17 (10)	5 (3)	10 (6)
Total Fortune 500	—	41 (64)	35 (54)	16 (24)	47 (76)	29 (47)	16 (26)	9 (15)
Plant Size—NJ								
001–199	42 (5)	23 (3)	8 (1)	0 (0)	69 (9)	31 (4)	0 (0)	0 (0)
200–499	40 (8)	23 (5)	18 (4)	23 (5)	73 (16)	9 (2)	0 (0)	18 (4)
500–5000	50 (8)	25 (4)	31 (5)	19 (3)	59 (10)	18 (3)	18 (3)	6 (1)
Company Size—NJ								
001–999	42 (5)	25 (3)	17 (2)	17 (2)	75 (9)	8 (1)	0 (0)	17 (2)
1000–2,999	36 (5)	33 (5)	13 (2)	7 (1)	68 (10)	20 (3)	7 (1)	7 (1)
3000–99998	58 (7)	15 (2)	23 (3)	31 (4)	69 (19)	8 (1)	8 (1)	15 (2)
Type of Industry—NJ								
Lo-Tech	39 (13)	27 (9)	24 (8)	21 (7)	68 (23)	12 (4)	3 (1)	18 (6)
Hi-Tech	44 (10)	21 (5)	13 (3)	8 (2)	67 (16)	25 (16)	8 (2)	0 (0)

* $P<.05$
** $P<.01$
*** $P<.001$

mitment of organizational resources, employee eligibility and participation, plans to start and expand programs, and exposure to planning and evaluation. The variable of organizational size, both plant size and company size, has been found to have a particularly strong impact on these and other aspects of worksite health promotion programs considered in this study.

Type of industry, measured here in terms of technological intensity, was also found to have some impact, though not nearly as much as size. It is possible that future research would demonstrate a greater impact for type of industry if the sample of organizations studied were to be expanded beyond manufacturing organizations to include those in other sectors, such as the information and service sectors. It is important, therefore, that the organizational characteristics of size and type of industry, among others, be taken into account whenever possible in studies of worksite health promotion.

A limitation of this study is its inability to distinguish levels of employee eligibility and participation for each health promotion activity. The failure to find differences in the rates of eligibility and participation by gender may, for example, be due in part to having asked about these issues as a whole, rather than for specific activities. Organizational characteristics such as size and type of industry are likely to assume even greater importance as studies begin to provide data on specific program activities. As certain health promotion activities emerge as central to programs in a given type of industry or industrial sector (such as accident prevention in the manufacturing sector, as documented here), future studies could focus on, and provide rich data about the nature of these activities.

The literature on worksite health promotion programs often cites improvement in employee health and cost savings as two of the major objectives of these programs. Given the centrality of these ideas in the literature, it was anticipated in this, and in the earlier study on the Fortune 500, that companies would employ formal planning, evaluation, and cost analysis techniques to develop and assess their programs. In fact, according to the findings from the two studies, most companies do not routinely adopt these techniques, and are particularly apt to forego cost analyses. This is of special interest when examined together with other findings on the high degree of organizational commitment of time and money for these programs. New Jersey respondents apparently shoulder a large share of costs (86% of all costs) and time burden. Without more planning, evaluation, and cost assessments, companies may be missing an opportunity to enhance the effectiveness of their programs. For example, the disparity found between the rates of employee eligibility and participation (about half of those eligible participate in programs) could be examined and addressed if planning methods, including needs assessments, were incorporated more fully into programs. Additionally, insufficient planning, evaluation, and cost analyses result in a lack of the necessary data against which to measure changes. These techniques along with organizational characteristics are likely to assume even greater importance as worksite health promotion programs evolve further to the point where they are fine-tuned to the unique requirements of particular types of organizational settings and participants.

REFERENCES

Chovil, A. C., Alexander, G. R., Gibson, J. J. & Altekruse, J. M. (1983). Occupational health services in South Carolina manufacturing plants: Results of a survey. *Public Health Reports, 98*(6), 597–603.

Danielson, D., & Danielson, K. (1980). *Ontario Employee Programme Survey.* Ministry of Culture and Recreation, Toronto.

Davis, L. (1982, October 18). A new definition of "high tech" reveals that U.S. competitiveness in this area is declining. *Business America, 18–23.*

Davis, M. F., Rosenberg, K., Iverson, D. C., Vernon, T. M., & Bauer, J. (1984). Worksite health promotion in Colorado. *Public Health Reports, 99,* 538–543.

Dean, P. J., Reid, L., & Gzowski, A. (1984). *A Planner's Guide to Fitness in the Workplace.* Ontario Ministry of Tourism and Recreation, Toronto.

Fielding, J. E., & Breslow, L. (1983). Health promotion programs sponsored by California employers. *American Journal of Public Health, 73,* 538–542.

Forouzesh, M. R., & Ratzker, L. E. (1984/1985). Health promotion and wellness programs: An insight into the Fortune 500. *Health Education, 15,* 18–22.

Freeman, C. (1982). *The Economics of Industrial Innovation.* Cambridge, Massachusetts: M.I.T. Press.

Herzlinger, R. E., & Calkins, D. (1986). How companies tackle health care costs: Part III. *Harvard Business Review, 64,* 70–80.

Hollander, R. B., & Lengermann, J. J. (1986). Fortune 500 companies: Long on wellness, short on evaluation. *Corporate Commentary, 2,* 51–52.

Hollander, R. B., & Lengermann, J. J. (1988). Corporate characteristics and worksite health promotion programs: Survey findings from Fortune 500 companies. *Social Science and Medicine. 26*(5), 491–501.

Hull, F., & Hage, J. (1980). A Prospectus for the 1980 Restudy of 110 New Jersey Factories. Technical Report #3, Research Program for Innovation and Productivity Strategies. New Brunswick, NJ: Rutgers University.

New Jersey Directory of Manufacturers (1984). Midland Park, NJ: Commerce Register, Inc.

Shain, M., Suurvali, H., & Boutilier, M. (1986). *Healthier Workers: Health Promotion and Employee Assistance Programs.* Lexington, MA: Lexington Books.

Shanklin, W. I., & Ryans, J. K. (1984). *Marketing High Technology.* Lexington, MA: Lexington Books.

Windom, R. E., McGinnis, J. M., & Fielding, J. E. (1987, July). Examining worksite health promotion. *Business and Health,* 36–37.

8

THE CAUSES AND SOLUTIONS TO OCCUPATIONAL INJURIES AMONG NURSES: AN ATTRIBUTIONAL STUDY

Suzanne Laidlaw Feldman

Robert H. L. Feldman

The causes and solutions to occupational injuries were examined among a sample of 93 hospital nurses. A personal-environmental perspective was utilized to determine nurses' perceptions of needle puncture injuries. The results of the study indicate that the nurse participants perceived the personal characteristics of the injured nurse as the most important factor in perceived responsibility for the injury, perceived cause of the injury, and perceived avoidance of the injury. Environmental factors were considered, but to a lesser degree. In terms of solutions to reducing needle injuries, the nurse participants judged environmentally oriented solutions as more effective than person-change solutions. Thus, by examining occupational injuries from the perspective of the individuals employed in the work environment, an alternative perspective is offered in the designing of effective occupational health programs.

The causes and solutions to occupational injuries have been analyzed from different perspectives. Some researchers have emphasized environmental factors, such as workplace conditions (Douglas, 1975; Samuels, 1974), while other investigators report personal factors such as attitudes, general behavior characteristics and personality of the worker as the main cause of occupational injuries (Schultz & Schultz, 1986; Verhagen, Vanhalst, Derijke, & Van Hoecke, 1976).

Hagglund (1976) conducted one of the few studies that empirically examined personal and environmental factors related to occupational injuries. A random sample of 257 injuries was selected from a collection of 2,610 postinjury investigation reports by the Wisconsin Safety and Building

Division. Hagglund found that 54% of the injuries were due to environmental factors (Wisconsin safety code violations or other unsafe working conditions), 35% were due to personal factors (the employee committed an unsafe act or made a mistake while working), 4% were due to both environmental and personal factors, and 7% had no clear indications of either factor.

Because of the complex nature of occupational injuries, safety behavior and occupational injuries need to be viewed in Lewinian terms (Lewin, 1936) as a function of both the person and the environment, that is, $B = f(P,E)$. The study described below examines occupational injuries among nurses in a hospital workplace from a personal-environmental perspective. That is, occupational injuries and solutions to reduce injuries are viewed as having both personal and environmental components.

Since the passage of the Occupational Safety and Health Act (OSHA) in 1970, increased interest has focused on the occupational injury rate in American industries including hospitals. A report by the National Institute for Occupational Safety and Health (NIOSH, 1974), the Hospital Occupational Health Services Study, concluded that the injury rate for hospitals, although not as high as the rates for heavy manufacturing or construction, did surpass the rates for many other industries, and had increased by almost 15% from 1958 to 1970. The occupational injury-illness rate for full-time private hospital workers was 8.8/1000 full-time workers. This rate was similar to the injury-illness rate of workers in agricultural production, electrical equipment manufacturing, and cigarette manufacturing. Among the most common injuries cited by the study were needle puncture injuries, back injuries, and sprains and strains.

Stellman, in an analysis of hospital working conditions, indicates that many different hazards exist in the hospital setting. These include contaminated needles, infections and parasitic diseases, toxic chemicals, ionizing radiation, anesthetic gasses, heavy lifting, heat, noise, electric equipment, dangerous patients, and a stressful environment (Stellman, 1978; Stellman & Snow, 1986). In addition, among the hospital staff, nurses have a greater likelihood of being exposed to these hazards and, therefore, of having higher rates of occupational-related illness and injuries. Lewy (1981) reported on a study at a major medical center that found that though nurses represented 33% of the hospital work force they accounted for 60% of the occupational injuries. Also, in an epidemiological study of hospital occupational injuries Braver (1978) found that the most common injury among hospital workers was needle puncture injuries among nurses. In Braver's study 18% of the hospital injuries were needle injuries among nurses. Therefore, to assist in the development of occupational safety programs to reduce needle puncture injuries among nurses the following study was conducted. The study's purpose was (a) to determine the cause(s) that nurses attribute to needle injuries—that is, what proportion do the nurses feel are due to personal factors of the injured party, and what proportion do they feel are due to environmental workplace conditions; and (b) to determine the solutions and strategies that nurses feel are most effective in reducing occupational injuries.

METHOD

Subjects

The subjects of the study were 93 nurses who were employed at a large urban hospital. The nurses were 92% female and 8% male. The age of the sample consisted of 88% under 25 years of age and 12% over 25 years of age. The educational level was 59% with bachelor's degree, 26% with nursing diplomas and 15% with associate degrees.

Materials

Based upon an epidemiological investigation of medical records and workers' compensation claims, as well as extensive conversations with hospital authorities, staff nurses, and safety officials, a list of factors contributing to needle injuries and a list of solutions to reduce occupational needle injuries were developed. From the lists three main factors were examined: personal characteristics of the injured nurse, environmental conditions of the workplace at the time of the injury, and severity of the injury. To determine how nurses perceived the causes and solutions to needle injuries, the nurses paticipating in this study received descriptions of needle injuries varying in terms of the personal characteristics of the nurse, the environmental workplace conditions, and the severity of the injury. Two levels of each factor were combined to form eight written descriptions of a needle injury in a Personal factor (2) × Environmental factors (2) × Severity of injury (2) design. The two levels of each factor were the personal characteristics of the nurse (either positive or negative), hospital environmental conditions (either positive or negative), and severity of the injury (either mild or severe).

The positive personal characteristics of the nurse included such items as no previous record of injuries and indication that the nurse was concentrating on what she was doing when the injury occurred. The negative personal characteristics indicated a previous record of injuries and indication that the nurse was not concentrating on what she as doing when the injury occurred.

The positive hospital environmental characteristics noted an ample supply of nurses on the floor at the time of the injury and an empty needle disposal unit. The negative hospital environmental characteristics mentioned a shortage of nurses on the floor at the time of the injury and a needle disposal unit that was filled to the very top. The mild injury was described as a needle that scratched the nurse's skin, whereas the severe injury was a dirty needle from a patient suspected of having hepatitis that penetrated the nurse's skin (Feldman, 1986).

The questionnaire consisted of two parts. The first part contained three items, each with its own scale. Item 1 was designed to measure how much the participants perceived the injured nurse to be responsible for the injury. The scale for this item varied from 1, not at all responsible, to 7, completely responsible. Item 2 was designed to measure how the participants perceived the cause of the injury in terms of personal and environmental factors. The scale varied from 1 (100% environmental factors/0% personal factors) to 11 (0% environmental factors/100% personal factors). Item 3 was designed to measure the paticipants' perception of whether the injured nurse could have avoided the needle injury. The scale varied from 1, definitely no, to 7, definitely yes.

Part two of the questionnaire consisted of a list of 10 solutions and strategies to reduce needle injuries. For each solution/strategy there was a seven-point scale, where 1 was not at all effective and 7 was extremely effective. The list of 10 solutions consisted of 5 personally-oriented solutions and 5 environmentally-oriented solutions that were listed in random order. The 5 personal-oriented solutions were talks and information, informational safety posters and newsletters, group discussions, rewards to individual nurses, and rewards to nursing stations. The 5 environment-oriented solutions were more inspections, more needle units, use of medication carts with disposal units on the carts, more frequent emptying of the disposal unit, and a needle disposal unit built into the wall in each patient's room. The list of solutions to reduce needle injuries was developed following extensive meetings and discussions with hospital nursing authorities, staff nurses, and hospital safety officials. For example, these experts suggested various changes in the use of disposal units as possible environmental solutions to reducing injuries. The goal in developing this list of solutions was to use those solutions that could actually be implemented.

Procedure

Each of the 93 nurses was randomly given a written description of one of the eight possible situations describing a needle injury. Each was asked to read the description carefully and complete the two part questionnaire.

RESULTS

Separate analyses of variance were conducted for each of the three dependent variables; that is, for perceived responsibility for the injury, perceived cause of the injury, and perceived avoidance of the injury. The independent variables, that is, the factors that varied in the descriptions, were personal factors, environmental factors, and severity. The analysis of variance for the responsibility variable revealed satistically significant main effects for the personal factor, $F(1,76) = 7.3$, $p<.01$ and the environmental factor, $F(1,76) = 6.0, p<.05$. No other effects or interactions were significant. Table 1 presents the means for these main effects. For personal factors, the nurse with negative characteristics, that is, the inattentive nurse, was perceived as more responsible for the injury than the attentive nurse, that is, the nurse with positive characteristics. The significant environmental main effect indicates that the nurse working in the negative hospital environment with the shortage of nurses was perceived as less responsible for the injury than the nurse who worked in a positive environment.

An analysis of the causality of the injury revealed significant main effects for personal factors, $F(1,76) = 13.4, p<.001$, and environmental factors, $F(1,76) = 6.0, p<.05$. The injury to the inattentive nurse was considered to be more the result of personal factors than the injury to the attentive nurse. The injury to the nurse in the negative hospital environment was attributed to environ-

TABLE 1
The Effect of Personal and Environmental Factors on Perceptions of Responsibility, Cause, and Avoidance of Needle Injuries

Independent Variables		Dependent Variables		
		Responsibility[1]	Cause[2]	Avoidance[3]
Person	Positive	4.1	5.4	4.8
	Negative	5.1**	7.1***	5.8***
Environment	Positive	5.0	6.8	5.3
	Negative	4.1*	5.7*	5.3

$*p < .05$ $**p < .01$ $***p < .001$

1. Responsibility was measured by a 7-point scale; the higher the number the more the nurse was perceived responsible for the injury.
2. Cause was measured by a 11-point scale; the higher the number the more that the personal factors of the nurse were perceived as the cause of the injury.
3. Avoidance was measured by a 7-point scale; the higher the number the more the nurse was perceived to be able to avoid the injury.

mental causes, whereas the injury to the nurse in the favorable hospital setting was attributed to personal causes (see Table 1).

An analysis of the third dependent measure, the avoidance of the injury, revealed a significant main effect for personal factors, $F(1,76) = 12.1, p<.001$, but no significant effect for environmental factors, $F(1,76) = <1$, n.s. The inattentive nurse was perceived as being able to avoid the injury more than the attentive nurse (see Table 1). In terms of severity of the needle injury the severe injury was perceived to be significantly more severe than the mild injury; however, severity of the injury did not influence perceptions of responsibility, causality, and avoidance.

To determine the relative importance of personal characteristics, environmental characteristics, and severity of the injury, on the three dependent measures, a canonical correlation analysis was conducted. Canonical correlation is a multivariate statistical technique that provides a means of identifying associations between sets of variables (Laessig & Duckett, 1979), in this case, the set of independent variables and the set of dependent variables. A statistical relationship was found between the two sets of variables, $\chi^2 (35) = 80.6, p<.001$. The independent variable, personal factor, was the only independent variable to have a heavy loading over .70; personal factors had a loading of .72. Therefore, of the three factors, the characteristics of the injured nurse—that is, personal factors—was the most important factor in making judgments about needle injuries.

Solutions to Reduce Injuries

Nurses' perceptions of the effectiveness of personal and environmental solutions to reduce needle injuries were also analyzed. The five environmental solutions as a group were considered more effective than the five personal solutions as a group as determined by a t-test ($t(92) = 8.6, p<.001$). The most effective solutions, according to the nurse participants, were more frequent inspections of disposal units and more frequent emptying of disposal units. Environmental solutions were considered more effective in reducing occupational injuries in the negative hospital environment than in the positive hospital environment. The least effective solutions were talks and information on preventing needle injuries and awards to individual nurses with good safety records. Personal solutions were considered especially ineffective for the attentive nurse with the mild needle injury.

DISCUSSION

The objective of the study was to determine which factors nurses perceive as important in their judgments of the causes and solutions to needle injuries.

To design an effective program to reduce injuries, it is important to determine the participants' perceptions of causes and solutions. Too often programs are designed without input from the recipients of the programs. The most common approach is to present information in the form of lectures and reading material at inservice classes called "generic safety education." Two underlying negative messages are sent to the participants. First, the participants are treated in a "passive manner." However, a key to effective safety education is active participation and input from the participants. Secondly, the focus of these programs is often on changing the behavior of the worker, and not on changing the environment, or changing both. Consequently, responsibility for causes and solutions is assumed to be attributed to the worker. In these typical inservice programs, therefore, there is a tendency to blame the victim—that is, the nurse—for the injury. Therefore, an inservice program may not be effective, because the goals of the program may not be perceived as relevant to the participants. Thus the participants may attribute the causes and solutions to different factors and believe that the program is not applicable to them.

The results of the present study indicate that personal characteristics of the injured nurse was the most important factor in judging injuries. The nurse described as having a previous record of injuries, and who was not concentrating when the injury occurred was considered more responsible for the injury than the nurse with the more positive characteristics. Personal factors were considered more important than environmental factors in determining causality of the injury, and it was generally felt that the injured nurse could have avoided the injury. However, although the nurses in this study considered the personal characteristics of the nurse the most important factor, they did not ignore environmental factors. Environmental factors were considered, but to a lesser degree than personal factors. What was most interesting about this factor was that if this nurse was injured in a positive hospital environment, then causality and responsibility were attributed to the nurse regardless of the nurse's actions. Coupled with the other findings about personal factors, one could interpret this finding to mean that nurses expect high standards of professional performance. They will attribute responsibility to themselves rather than to other factors, unless it is clearly indicated that environmental factors are involved.

Although personal characteristics were viewed as more important than environmental characteristics in determining the cause of needle injuries, environmental solutions were judged more effective in reducing these injuries than personal solutions. In fact, the top four solutions to reducing injuries all supported changes in the hospital working environment (a replication of this study in a second hospital revealed similar trends for perceptions of causes and solutions; Feldman, 1986). This difference between perceived causes and perceived solutions may appear to be contradictory. One explanation is that even if one perceives personal factors as the cause of injuries, the best approach may be to alter the workplace environment rather than attempt to change personal behavior. This approach to occupational injuries is similar to Haddan and Baker (1978), who assert that whatever the contribution of personal factors to injuries, effective preventive strategies should utilize "passive" environmental measures that do not require the individual to take some specific action to avoid injuries. However, as previously stated, many hospital programs to reduce occupational injuries among nurses utilize talks, informational and inservice classes—that is, the solution perceived least effective among the nurses in this study.

In the present study, nurses evaluated "vignettes" that were developed after discussions with nurses and administrators. In these vignettes, when the work environment was negative, nurses attributed the causes and solutions to the environment rather than to the personal factors of nurses in the vignettes. Further research is needed, to determine how nurses perceive their actual "work environment."

Recently, with the shortage of nurses in hospital settings, nurses responsible for more patients, demands for working overtime increasing, fears of contracting AIDS and fears of malpractice suits, many nurses perceive their work environments as negative. It is possible that those negative perceptions are so pervasive that individuals are not even entering this occupational field, or if they do become nurses they are choosing nonhospital settings.

If this is true, then new approaches to reduce occupational injuries among nurses are needed. The results of this study indicate that hospital nurses believe that environmental workplace changes are needed to solve this problem. Therefore, there is a need to restructure safety programs from a person-environment perspective. First, assessment is needed to determine how nurses perceive their actual work environment. Secondly, changes in the work environment need to be made. The message to be given to workers is that the administration is responsive to the worker. Therefore, by investigating the perceptions of hospital nurses, a new approach to the development of ocupational health programs is offered.

REFERENCES

Braver, E. (1978). *Hospital occupational safety and health: A medical record study of housekeepers and a study of workers' compensation claims of hospital employees at a large university hospital.* Unpublished manuscript, Johns Hopkins University.

Douglas, B. E. (1975). Occupation health problems in clinics and hospitals. In C. Zenz (Ed.), *Occupational medicine: Principles and practical applications.* Chicago: Year Book Medical Publishers.

Feldman, R.H.L. (1986). Hospital injuries. *Occupational Health and Safety, 55*(9), 12–15.

Haddan, W., & Baker, S. P. (1978). Injury control. In D. Clark & B. MacMahon (Eds., 2nd ed.), *Preventive medicine.* Boston: Little Brown and Company.

Hagglund, G. (1976). *OSHA: Causes of injury in industry—The "unsafe act" theory.* Madison, Wisconsin: University of Wisconsin Extension School for Workers. Laessig, R. E., & Duckett, E. J. (1979). Canonical correlation analysis: Potential for environmental health planning. *American Journal of Public Health, 69,* 353–359.

Lewin, K. (1936). *Principles of topological psychology.* New York: McGraw-Hill.

Lewy, R. (1981). Prevention strategies in hospital occupational medicine. *Journal of Occupational Medicine, 23,* 109–111.

NIOSH (1974). *Hospital Occupational Health Services Study* (Vol. 1, Publication No. 75–101). Washington, DC: National Institute for Occupational Safety and Health (HEW).

Samuels, S. W. (1974). Behavioral Science and occupational health. In C. Xinteras, B. L. Johnson, & I. DeGrant (Eds.), *Behavioral toxicology: Early detection of occupational hazards.* Washington, DC: National Institute for Occupational Safety and Health.

Schultz, D. P., & Schultz, S. E. (1986). *Psychology and industry today* (4th ed.). New York: Macmillan.

Stellman, J. M. (1978). *Women's work, women's health: Myths and realities.* New York: Pantheon.

Stellman, J. M., & Snow, B. R. (1986). Occupational safety and health hazards and the psychosocial health and well-being of workers. In M. F. Cataldo & T. J. Coates (Eds.), *Health and industry: A behavioral medicine perspective.* New York: John Wiley.

Verhagen, P., Vanhalst, B., Derijcke, H., & Van Hoecke, M. (1976). The value of same psychological theories on industrial accidents. *Journal of Occupational Accidents, 1,* 39–45.

9

HEALTH LOCUS OF CONTROL IN THE HOSPITAL: HOSPITAL WORKERS' BELIEFS ABOUT CONTROL OVER INJURIES

Robert H. L. Feldman

Suzanne Laidlaw Feldman

The Multidimensional Health Locus of Control Scales were expanded to include a fourth dimension: environment locus of control, the belief that environmental conditions control one's health. The expanded scales were utilized in an investigation of needle injuries among hospital nurses. Thus, Needle Injury Locus of Control (NI-LOC) Scales were used to determine hospital nurses' beliefs about control over needle injuries. The findings of the study indicate that hospital nurses were strongly internally oriented, moderately environmentally-oriented, and weakly powerful-other and chance oriented. In addition, the four dimensions were significantly related to perceptions about the causes and solutions to needle injuries, therefore giving support to the construct validity of the measures. The results of the investigation indicate that the addition of an environmental dimension improves our understanding of health behavior, especially in workplace settings.

Health locus of control measures the extent to which individuals perceive that they have control over their health (Wallston & Wallston, 1978). Health locus of control scales have been utilized in school settings (Noland, Riggs, & Hall, 1987; Parcel & Meyers, 1978), in community settings (Noland & Feldman, 1985; Wallston, Wallston & DeVellis, 1978), and among patient populations (Lewis, Morisky, & Flynn, 1978; Meyers, Donham, & Ludenia, 1982). However, little research has examined health locus of control in work settings. Employees in work settings are frequently exposed to a variety of workplace hazards, such as toxic chemicals, radiation, and occupational stressors. The question then arises as to whether workers perceive that they have control over their health and safety in this environmental setting; that is, are they "internally-oriented," believing that they have control over their health and safety; "powerful other-oriented," believing that powerful others, such as their supervisors, control their health and safety; or "chance-oriented," believing that chance, fate, or luck control their health and safety.

In the workplace setting, environmental conditions may affect locus of control in still another way. Feldman and Feldman (1989, this volume) point out that perception of occupational injuries is a function of both personal acts and environmental conditions. Workers exposed to unsafe workplace conditions are likely to attribute their injuries or illnesses to the workplace environment. Thus, a fourth orientation that workers could have is an "environmental-orientation," which is the belief that environmental work-place conditions control their health and safety. The environmental locus of control is another dimension of the external locus of control. If individuals believe that they themselves do not control their health (i.e., they are not internal), then they are externally-oriented. They believe that (a) powerful others, (b) chance, fate or luck, and/or (c) environmental conditions affect their health and safety.

The environmental-orientation is especially relevant to the workplace. However, Noland and Feldman (1984, 1985) utilized an environmental locus of control scale in their study of exercise behavior among adult women. They developed an Exercise Locus of Control Scale, which measured an individual's control over her exercise behavior. This scale had four subscales, which included one internal and three external scales (powerful others, chance, and environment). The environmental scale included factors such as weather and the availability of equipment, as they relate to control of exercise behavior. Therefore, the addition of a fourth dimension to the multidimentional health locus of control expands and adds greater specificity to the scale.

Rotter (1975) and Wallston and Wallston (1981) recommend the use of greater specificity to improve the validity of the locus of control measures. Specificity can be increased by using a scale specific to the behavior under investigation rather than using a generalized health locus of control scale. In the following study we examined occupational injuries common to the hospital workplace setting. In particular, health locus of control concerning needle puncture injuries, a common occupational injury, was investigated (Braver, 1978; NIOSH, 1974). To determine whether hospital nurses perceive that they have control over needle injuries, a Needle Injury Locus of Control (NI-LOC) scale was developed. This multidimensional health locus of control scale consisted of four subscales, one internal and three external. The scales were (a) internal, (b) powerful other, (c) chance, and (d) environment. Thus the NI-LOC Scale was more specific in two ways. First, it consist of four dimensions, and second, the scale was specific to needle injuries.

METHOD

Subjects

A sample of 93 nurses employed at a large urban hospital participated in the study. The sample was 91% female and 8% male.

Materials

A questionnaire was developed to measure hospital nurses' locus of control in terms of needle injuries. Four scales were developed: (a) internal NI-LOC, (b) powerful-others NI-LOC, (c) chance NI-LOC, and (d) environment NI-LOC (see Table 1). The NI-LOC scale items were mixed with generalized LOC scale items and health LOC scale items. All items utilized a 5-point Likert format, with "strongly agree" scored as five, "agree" as four, "uncertain" as three, "disagree" as two, and "strongly disagree" as one.

In addition, the participants received descriptions of needle injuries. They were asked to determine responsibility for the needle injuries, measured on a 7-point scale, the cause of the needle injuries in terms of personal and environmental factors measured on an 11-point scale; and whether the needle injuries could have been avoided, measured on a 7-point scale. Also, the subjects were given a list of 10 solutions to reduce needle injuries consisting of 5 personally-oriented and 5 environmentally-oriented solutions in random order. For each solution they were asked to evaluate its effectiveness on a 7-point scale (Feldman & Feldman, 1989, this volume).

RESULTS

Descriptive information for the Needle Injury Locus of Control Scale (NI-LOC) and additional scales is provided in Table 2. Since each NI-LOC dimension consisted of three items, these items were summed to form four dimensions. Using a 5-point Likert scale, the possible range of each NI-LOC dimension was 3 to 15, with an expected mean value of 9. To determine how the NI-LOC scales compared with more traditional scales, Health Locus of Control (H-LOC) items from Wallston, Wallston, and DeVellis (1978) and

TABLE 1
Needle Injury Locus of Control Scale

Internal (NI-LOC)
27. The main thing that affects whether I get a needle injury is what I do myself.
30. If I take the right actions I can avoid needle injuries.
35. Whether or not I have a needle injury depends mostly on how careful I am.

Powerful Others (NI-LOC)
26. Following my supervisor's orders to the letter is the best way to avoid a needle injury.
29. I can only avoid needle injuries with the help of hospital administrators.
32. Whether or not I have a needle injury depends mostly on other people.

Chance (NI-LOC)
19. If it's meant to be, I will have a needle injury.
21. No matter what I do, if I am going to have a needle injury, I will have a needle injury.
24. Whether or not I have a needle injury is mostly a matter of luck.

Environment (NI-LOC)
18. The workplace environment plays a big part in whether I have a needle injury or not.
33. If the workplace environment is designed properly then I will not have needle injuries.
37. Whether or not I have a needle injury is determined by the workplace environment.

Generalized Locus of Control (G-LOC) items were included with the NI-LOC items. Since only one H-LOC items was used for each dimension, that item score was weighted by a multiple of 3. Similarly, two items were used with each dimension of the G-LOC; therefore, each two-item dimension score was weighted by a factor of 1.5.

The results in Table 2 indicate that the hospital nurses have a strong internal orientation in terms of needed injuries. Inasmuch as 9 is the expected mean value and 15 is the maximum possible score, a score of 12.7 indicates a substantial internal locus of control orientation.

In terms of the external dimensions, the strongest dimension was the environmental locus of control. A score of 8.5 was close to the mean value, therefore indicating an intermediate environmental orientation. That is, the nurses perceived that the environment plays a moderate role in whether they have a needle injury. Both the powerful others dimension and the chance dimension produced low scores, 5.5 and 5.1, respectively. Therefore, the hospital nurses were highly internally-oriented, moderately environmental-

TABLE 2
Descriptive Data on Scales

Locus of Control	Scale[1] NI-LOC[2,3]	H-LOC[4]	G-LOC[5]
Internal	12.7 (2.1)	12.9	12.8
Powerful others	5.5 (1.7)	7.8	6.3
Chance	5.1 (2.2)	5.4	5.6
Environment	8.5 (2.5)	9.0	8.1

[1]Mean values
[2]NI-LOC, Needle Injury Locus of Control
[3]( )— Standard deviation
[4]H-LOC, Health Locus of Control, weighted values
[5]G-LOC, General Locus of Control, weighted values

ly-oriented, and low in terms of powerful others and chance. Also, it should be noted that Health Locus of Control Scores and Generalized Locus of Control Scores showed similar results (see Table 2).

In Tables 3 and 4 the intercorrelations between NI-LOC scales and H-LOC scales and G-LOC scales are presented. Generally, each multidimensional scale correlated highly with its theoretical counterpart. For example, C-NILOC scale correlated, $r = .59$, with C-HLOC scale; the E-NILOC scale correlated, $r = .44$, with E-HLOC; the C-NILOC correlated $r = .53$ with C-GLOC scale; and E-NILOC scale correlated, $r = .47$, with E-GLOC scale. Also, in general, the internal scales correlate negatively with the three external scales.

TABLE 3
Intercorrelations of NI-LOC Scales and H-LOC Scales

	I-NILOC	P-NILOC	C-NILOC	E-NILOC
I-NILOC				
P-NILOC	−.49	—		
C-NILOC	−.44	.33	—	
E-NILOC	−.30	.38	.12	—
I-HLOC	.29	−.31	−.25	−.11
P-HLOC	.03	.15	−.02	.04
C-HLOC	−.31	.22	.59	.14
E-HLOC	−.32	.35	.13	.44

For N = 93,
$r = .17\ p < .05$
$r = .24\ p < .01$
$r = .31\ p < .001$

TABLE 4
Intercorrelations of NI-LOC Scales and G-LOC Scales

	I-NILOC	P-NILOC	C-NILOC	E-NILOC
I-GLOC	.52	-.50	-.49	-.21
P-GLOC	-.47	.54	.25	.35
C-GLOC	-.50	.56	.53	.23
E-GLOC	-.31	.35	.22	.47

For N = 93,
$r = .17\, p < .05$
$r = .24\, p < .01$
$r = .31\, p < .001$

To determine the construct validity of NI-LOC scales, correlations were computed between the NI-LOC scale and the causes and solutions to reduce needle injuries. In Table 5, correlations between responsibility, cause, and avoidance of needle injuries and the NI-LOC Scales are presented. The results indicate the more internal-oriented the nurse the more she felt that nurses were responsible for needle injuries ($r = .22, p < .05$). In contrast, the more environmentall-oriented the nurse, the more she felt that nurses were not responsible for needle injuries ($r = -.25, p < .01$), but that environmental factors were the cause of the injuries ($r = .31, p < .01$). In terms of the avoidance of needle injuries, the more internal-oriented the nurse, the more she felt that injuries could be avoided ($r = .37, p < .001$); while the more chance-oriented the nurse the more she felt that injuries could not be avoided ($r = -.24, p < .01$).

An examination of the correlations between the NI-LOC scales and the solutions to reduce needle injuries gave further support to the construct validity of the NI-LOC scales (Table 6). A significant correlation was found

TABLE 5
Intercorrelations of NI-LOC Scales with Responsibility, Cause, and Avoidance of Needle Injuries

	Responsibility	Cause	Avoidance
I-NILOC	.22*	-.10	.37***
P-NILOC	-.17	.11	-.14
C-NILOC	-.05	.13	-.24**
E-NILOC	-.25**	.31**	-.17

$* p < .05$
$** p < .01$
$*** p < .001$

TABLE 6
Intercorrelations of NI-LOC Scales with Solutions to Reduce Needle Injuries

	P (Total)[1]	P1	P2	P3	P4	P5
I-NILOC	.19*	.07	.18*	.18*	.07	.22*
P-NILOC	.09	−.03	.06	.11	.15	.05
C-NILOC	−.06	−.07	−.06	−.02	.01	−.05
E-NILOC	−.05	−.01	−.09	.05	.09	−.03
	E (Total)[2]	E1	E2	E3	E4	E5
I-NILOC	−.09	−.10	−.03	.10	−.17	−.09
P-NILOC	.10	.09	.10	−.01	.04	.18*
C-NILOC	−.09	−.03	−.09	−.24**	.06	−.02
E-NILOC	.18*	.02	.21*	.14	.07	.21*

* $p < .05$
** $p < .01$
[1]P—Personal change solutions
[2]E—Environmental change solutions

between an internal orientation (I-NILOC scores) and perceptions that person change solutions (in general) are an effective means to reduce needle injuries ($r = .19$, $p < .05$). Also, a significant correlation was reported between an environmental orientation (E-NILOC scores) and the belief that environmental change solutions (in general) are an effective means to reduce needle injuries ($r = .18$, $p < .05$).

In terms of specific solutions to reduce needle injuries, three out of the five person-change solutions were significantly correlated with an internal orientation. None of the external orientations were related to the belief that person change solutions are an effective approach to reduce needle injuries. In terms of the environmental change solutions, two out of five solutions were related to an environmental orientation. Also, specific environmental solutions were correlated with the two other external orientations, powerful others, and chance.

DISCUSSION

The workplace offers health educators unique opportunities to expand the empirical base of health education, to increase the generalizability of findings, and to examine variables specific to worksettings (Hollander & Feldman, 1986). Since health locus of control researchers have virtually ignored the workplace, it is useful to determine how workers perceive their control over health and safety in this environmental setting. The workplace is a setting in which environmental conditions can affect one's health and safety. Therefore, an environmental dimension was added to the Multidimensional Health Locus of Control Scale. Since greater specificity may improve the validity of locus of control scales, scales specific to a workplace situation were developed. In this study, a needle injury locus of control (NI-LOC) scale was developed. The results of this study indicate that in terms of needle injuries hospital nurses were strongly internally-oriented, moderately environmental-ly-oriented, and weakly powerful other and chance oriented. Thus, the addition of a fourth health locus of control dimension, the environmental dimension, increases our knowledge of how nurses perceive their health and safety.

Comparisons of the NI-LOC Scales and the Multidimensional H-LOC and G-LOC indicate strong to moderate correlations between similar constructs for almost all scales (only the correlation between P-NILOC and P-HLOC was nonsignificant). This gives support to the theoretical soundness of these scales. Additional support for the NI-LOC Scales is given from the intercorre-lations between the NI-LOC Scales and the causes and solutions to needle injuries. The more internal-oriented the nurse, the more she felt that nurses were responsible for needle injuries, that nurses cause these injuries, and that the best solutions to reduce injuries were person-change solutions. In contrast, the more environment-oriented the nurse, the more she felt that nurses were not responsible for needle injuries, that environmental conditions were the cause of injuries, and that the best solutions were to change the hospital workplace environment.

The results of this study give support to the usefulness of the environmental locus of control as an external dimension. The other external dimensions, powerful others and chance, exhibited few significant correlations, and most of these were lower in magnitude in comparison to the environmental locus of control. Thus, in the workplace situation, without the environmental dimension we would be missing valuable information. Noland and Feldman's (1984) study of exercise behavior also found the environmental dimension to be essential. The only locus of control scale to correlate with exercise behavior was the environmental scale ($r = -.33, p <$ .01). The greater the belief that environmental factors (e.g., weather, equipment) controlled their exercise behavior, the less the women participants exercised.

It is argued that when designing a safety and health education program, both personal and environmental factors need to be considered (see Feldman and Feldman, 1989, this volume). Inservice programs are often presented from an authoritarian perspective; that is, workers are directed to change their behavior by administrators or "powerful others." The results of this study suggest that directing behavior change by powerful others, without considering changes in the environment and without considering the health locus of control of the participants may not be effective. It is recommended that safety and health inservice programs need to be designed from the perspective of the participants with consideration of factors such as locus of control, that is, participatory safety health education rather than an imposed authoritarian perspective. Emphasis should be placed on how nurses can "control" or change their environment.

In conclusion, in many settings, such as work places, outdoor leisure activities, and patient settings, environmental factors play an important role. The addition of an environmental scale to the Multidimensional Health Locus of Control Scale can improve our understanding of health behavior in these settings.

REFERENCES

Braver, E. (1978). *Hospital occupational safety and health: A medical record study of housekeepers and a study of workers' compensation claims of hospital employees at a large university hospital.* Unpublished manuscript, Johns Hopkins University.

Feldman, S. L., & Feldman, R.H.L. (1989). The causes and solutions to occupational injuries among nurses: An attributional study. In R.H.L. Feldman & J. H. Humphrey (Eds.), *Advances in Health Education: Current Research, Vol. 2* (pp. 117–125). New York: AMS Press.

Hollander, R. B., & Feldman, R.H.L. (1986). Health education research in the workplace. *Health Education, 17*(3), 34–37.

Lewis, F. M., Morisky, D. E., & Flynn, B. S. (1978). A test of the construct validity of health locus of control: Effects on self-reported compliance for hypertensive patients. *Health Education Monographs, 6*(1), 138–148.

Meyers, R., Donham, G. W., & Ludenia, K. (1982). The psychometric properties of the health locus of control scales with medical and surgical patients. *Journal of Clinical Psychology, 38*(4), 783–787.

NIOSH (1974). *Hospital occupational health services study* (Vol. 1, Publication, 75–101. Washington, DC: National Institute for Occupational Safety and Health (HEW).

Noland, M. P., & Feldman, R.H.L. (1984) Factors related to the leisure exercise behavior of "returning" women college students. *Health Education 15*(2), 32–36.

Noland, M. P., & Feldman, R.H.L. (1985). An empirical investigation of leisure exercise behavior in adult women. *Health Education, 16*(5), 29–34.

Noland, M. P., Riggs, R. S., & Hall, J. W. (1987). A descriptive study of health locus of control and health status in secondary special education students. *Health Education, 18*(4), 8–13.

Parcel, G. S., & Meyers, M. P. (1978). Development of an instrument to measure children's health locus of control. *Health Education Monographs, 6*(1), 149–159.

Rotter, J. B. (1975). Some problems and misconceptions related to the construct of internal versus external control of reinforcement. *Journal of Consulting and Clinical Psychology, 43*, 56–67.

Wallston, B. S., & Wallston, K. A. (1978). Locus of control and health: A review of the literature. *Health Education Monographs, 6*(1), 107–117.

Wallston, K. A., & Wallston, B. S. (1981). Health locus of control scales. In H. Lefcourt (Ed.), *Research with the locus of control construct (Vol. 1)*. New York: Academic Press.

Wallston, K. A., Wallston, B. S., & DeVillis, R. (1978). Development of the multidimensional health locus of control (MHLC) scales. *Health Education Monographs, 6*(1), 160–170.

10

A SURVEY OF FIRE PROTECTIVE BEHAVIORS AND BELIEFS IN A COLLEGE POPULATION

Kenneth H. Beck

An anonymous survey questionnaire was administered to over 900 college students to measure their current fire protective behaviors and beliefs. The results revealed that active fire protective behavior is being practiced by only a minority of college students. Less than 20% of the sample reported performing an inspection of their home for fire hazards, practicing an emergency escape from their home, or vacuuming the dust from their smoke detector in the last six months. Forty percent or less reported having ever changed the batteries in their smoke detector, having the local number of the local emergency telephone number posted near their phone, and having a fire extinguisher in their home or ever using one. Most students (75%) actually knew the local emergency number and half had checked to see if their smoke detector was working within the last six months. Females were more likely to have practiced emergency escape whereas males were more likely to have practiced using a fire extinguisher. The belief data indicated that the sample did not feel particularly susceptible to fire hazards, but that females view the seriousness of fire hazards as greater than males, and their personal efficacy at controlling them as less than males. Females also view the effectiveness of various protective measures as greater than males.

Fires are a major cause of accidental death and disability in this country. According to the National Safety Council (1986), almost five thousand people died in fire-related incidents in 1985, making it the second leading cause of death in the home, behind falls. Fire losses totaled over $7 billion last year. The number of people who are injured but not killed each year in fires probably approaches several hundred thousand. Yet, despite the enormity of this national safety problem, there is surprisingly little research published in the area of public attitudes and practices regarding fire safety. However, there is a wealth of information available about the dynamics of human behavior in actual fire situations (e.g., Bryan, 1983, Keating, 1982, Paulsen, 1984), although little that pertains to human behavior before involvement in a fire event has taken place. The purpose of this paper is to present the results of a college campus survey of fire protective behaviors and beliefs.

There are several reasons for conducting a survey of college students regarding fire safety. First, these people often are at increased risk for fire incidents due to their lifestyle (e.g., smoking, excessive alcohol consumption, etc.), living arrangements (e.g., overcrowded apartments, high-rise dormitories, etc.), and their youthful exuberance may predispose them to feel either immune to the hazards of fire situations or overconfident at being able to handle them and protect themselves adequately from harm. Secondly, college students undoubtedly reflect the attitudes of society at large and thus mirror, to a certain extent, the values of a broad segment of the population. Finally, campus safety programs need to be responsive to the needs of their primary constituency (students), and without primary data on the perceptions of their target audience they will have no way of knowing if they are meeting their prevention goals and objectives.

METHOD

Sample. An anonymous questionnaire was developed and administered to over 1,000 college students attending various health education classes at the main campus of the University of Maryland. A total of 991 usable questionnaires were returned. The sample ranged in age from 17 to 67, with a mean of 21.13 years (SD = 4.01). There were 402 males (40.6%) and 582 females (58.7%) and 7 people that did not indicate their gender. There were 157 freshmen (15.8%), 282 sophomores (28.5%), 203 juniors (20.5%), and 349 seniors (35.2%). The sample appears to be slightly biased toward upper-level students and females. Therefore, the reader is urged to bear this in mind when interpreting the results.

An attempt was made to sample from as wide a variety of health classes as possible, so as to include a broad segment of the campus community. Within this university many health education courses enjoy a wide cross-campus appeal, and therefore attract students from a variety of majors, who take these courses for satisfying elective requirements. Since the number of registered health education majors at the time this survey was conducted was about 40, it seems reasonable to conclude that this sample was not predominantly biased with students whose primary major was health related. A decision was made not to sample from those classes (e.g., "Safety Education," "Behavioral Factors in Accident Causation and Prevention," etc.) that were primarily safety oriented. The types of classes sampled and their frequency are presented in Table 1.

Questionnaire. An anonymous questionnaire was developed to measure several aspects of fire safety. The items pertinent to this investigation dealt with the students' fire protective behaviors and beliefs. The first set of items concerned whether or not they had engaged in or experienced 13 separate fire-related behaviors, ranging from having changed the batteries in their smoke detector in the past year to ever having practiced an emergency escape from their home. All questions were worded in the same form as presented in Table 2. They all had "yes" or "no" response choices.

The second set of items were worded to reflect measures of the students' beliefs about fire safety. There were four types of beliefs, each of which was measured by four separate items (see Table 3). The first set of four items was designed to measure feelings of *vulnerability* or susceptibility to fires and fire hazards, and included such items as "How likely is it that there are significant fire hazards where you live?" All items were followed by a 5-point scale ranging from "Not at all likely" (scored as 1) to "Extremely likely" (scored as 5). The next set of items were designed to measure feelings of *seriousness* of fire hazards and included items such as "How concerned or worried are you about fire hazards that you know of in your home or where you live?" These were also followed by a 5-point scale ranging from "Not at all worried" (scored as 1) to Extremely worried" (scored as 5). The next set of four items were designed to measure the student's *personal efficacy* or adequacy of engaging in fire protective behavior, and included such items as "If a fire did break out in your home or place where you live, how effective do you think you would be in controlling it?" The same 5-point scale was used for these

TABLE 1
Frequency Distribution of Various Health Education Classes Used For Obtaining Sample

Health Education Class	Frequency	Percentage
Drug Use and Abuse	31	3.1
Personal & Community Health	36	3.6
First Aid & Emergency Service	57	5.8
Control Stress & Tension	425	42.9
Health Problems of Children & Youth	22	2.2
Women's Health	74	7.5
Death Education	82	8.3
Human Sexuality	235	23.7
Special Topics in Health	29	2.9

items as well. The final set of items were designed to measure the student's perceived *effectiveness* of various fire-protective behaviors (emergency escape planning, emergency escape practice, home fire safety inspections, and smoke detectors) at being able to prevent a fire from happening or protect them in the event of an actual fire situation. These were worded in the same way as the previous items (e.g., "How effective do you think emergency escape practice is at being able to protect you from being caught in a fire situation?"). The same 5-point response scale was used with these items.

RESULTS

The frequency analysis of the fire protective behaviors is presented in Table 2. These results revealed that less than half the sample had changed the batteries in their smoke detector (if they owned a battery operated detector) or vacuumed the dust from it, and that about half the sample had ever checked to see if it was in proper working order within the last six months. Only about 20% appeared to have performed an inspection of their home for fire hazards. About 80% reported that they knew the local emergency

TABLE 2
Frequency of Fire Protective Behaviors

Percentage Who:	Total Sample	Males	Females
Changed batteries in smoke detector last year	35.6	32.8	37.3
Checked to see if smoke detector was working in last six months	51.3	53.5	49.7
Vacuumed dust from smoke detector in last six months	10.0	8.2	10.7
Performed a fire inspection of their home for potential fire hazards	19.8	23.1	17.5
Reported to know the local emergency number	81.1	79.9	82.0
Actually knew the local emergency number	75.2	72.4	77.0
Had the local emergency number posted near their phone	37.4	40.5	35.1
Have ever practiced an emergency escape from their home	19.9	12.9	24.7
Have ever had a fire in their home	12.6	13.7	11.9
Have ever called the fire department	20.9	21.1	20.6
Have a fire extinguisher in their home	41.7	41.8	41.8
Know how to use it	52.2	67.7	41.6
Have ever tried to use a fire extinguisher	35.4	58.2	19.9

telephone number, however only 75% actually gave the correct number on the questionnaire, and only 37% had this number posted near their phone. Slightly less than 20% reported ever having practiced an emergency escape from their home, although females (24.7%) appear twice as likely to do so than males (12.9%). Approximately 12% reported ever having a fire in their home and 20% had called the fire department. Forty percent indicated there was a fire extinguisher in their home and 52% reported they knew how to use it, but only 35% reported that they have ever tried to use it. Females (41.6%) appear far less likely than males (67.7%) in knowing how to use a fire extinguisher and in ever using one (19.9% vs. 58.2%).

The next analysis performed was of the various belief measures. The mean for each item is presented in Table 3 for the entire sample and separately for

TABLE 3
Mean Fire Safety Beliefs

	Total Sample	Males	Females
Susceptibility (Alpha = .79)			
Likelihood of significant hazards	2.52	2.48	2.56
Unintended fire will start in home	2.02	2.06	2.12
Unintended fire will start in future	2.23	2.26	2.21
Involved in serious fire situations in future	1.97	2.05	1.92
Seriousness (Alpha = .79)			
Fire hazards in your home	2.11	2.03	2.16
Home might not be safe	2.08	1.98	2.15
Ever think about getting caught in a fire	2.34	2.09	2.52
Dangerousness of fire in your home	3.03	2.94	3.10
Personal Efficacy (Alpha = .83)			
If a fire did occur, how effective would you be at controlling it?	2.73	2.88	2.62
If a fire did occur, how effective would you be in knowing what to do	3.14	3.41	2.96
How adequate is your fire knowledge?	2.97	3.17	2.83
How competent do you think you would be in a fire situation?	3.03	3.31	2.84
Response Efficacy (Alpha = .73)			
How effective is/are:			
Emergency Escape Planning	3.46	3.33	3.55
Emergency Escape Practice	3.36	3.17	3.48
Fire Safety Inspections	3.57	3.49	3.62
Smoke Detectors	3.78	3.81	3.76

1–5 scale; 1 = not at all, 2 = slightly, 3 = moderately, 4 = very, 5 = extremely.

males and females. Inasmuch as the items within each belief set (i.e., susceptibility) were significantly ($p < .001$) intercorrelated, the four items in each set were summed to form a scale score and the males and females were compared. The alpha reliability coefficients of these scales were in excess of .70 (see Table 3). The means for the individual belief items are also presented in Table 3 for the entire sample and separately for males and females.

The males and females did not differ significantly on their feelings of susceptibility to fire threats. However they did differ on the other three beliefs. Males ($M = 8.98$) rated fire hazards as less serious than females ($M = 9.89$), $F(1,969) = 20.53$, $p < .001$; they rated their personal efficacy at controlling fire hazards ($M = 12.66$) higher than females ($M = 11.18$), $F(1,971) = 59.17$, $p < .001$; and they rated the effectiveness of the various protective activities ($M = 13.70$) lower than the females ($M = 14.36$), $F(1,963) = 11.84$, $p < .001$.

DISCUSSION

The results of this survey revealed that most college students in this sample are not actively involved in fire safety activities. Only about one half of the sample had checked their smoke detector in the last six months. Fewer still had engaged in other active fire protective measures. The most frequently observed phenomenon was knowledge of the local emergency telephone number. These findings are disturbing in that they suggest a tendency on the part of these students to rely upon passive (telephone for assistance) as opposed to active (inspecting home for fire hazards, practicing emergency escape) means of protecting themselves from fire. This is regrettable because the students are not adept in those activities that seem to be vital for their survival in the event of an actual fire.

Given the low frequency with which serious or life threatening fires occur on campus, it is understandable that many students may feel immune to them, or at least not consider fire hazards as highly salient. The belief data indicate

TABLE 4
Mean Scores on Fire Safety Belief Scales

	Susceptibility	Severity	Personal Efficacy	Response Efficacy
Males	8.77	8.98	12.66	13.70
Females	8.76	9.89	11.18	14.36

Note: Scale scores range from 4 (low) to 20 (high).

that most students perceive their susceptibility to fires (or at least being involved in a serious fire situation at some time in the future) as relatively low. This lack of perceived vulnerability may account for the low percentage of students who engaged in active prevention efforts.

What is surprising is the apparent lack of correspondence between the students' relatively strong beliefs in the effectiveness of such actions and their performance of these actions. The efficacy of all four actions (emergency escape planning, practice, fire safety inspections, and smoke detectors) were rated the highest among the entire set of belief items. Thus, convincing people of the adequacy of such measures does not seem to be the primary task of campus fire safety educators. What does seem to at issue here is convincing people of their vulnerability to these hazards as well as of their personal efficacy at fire protection.

Personal or self-efficacy has long been considered essential in initiating and sustaining threat-coping behavior (Bandura, 1977; 1982, 1986). These results indicate that whereas the overall level of reported personal efficacy appears to be at an adequate level, females may be in more need of personal efficacy-enhancing exercises than males. Females doubt their ability to handle a fire situation effectively in comparison with males. Although such differences are undoubtedly due to a variety of factors, it seems likely that this group is being underserved in terms of fire safety education. Therefore, future efforts on campus must target females as well as males and convince them of their capabilities in fire situations.

The implications of these initial survey results suggest that fire prevention on campus is not a particularly salient or important topic for most of the student community. Active fire protection seems to have been relegated to others (campus safety officials, fire department, emergency personnel, etc.) and is not performed by a majority of people. Therefore, the primary tasks of campus fire safety professionals are to communicate effectively the importance of active and preventive fire protection measures to this population, provide the necessary skill training in performing these activities effectively, especially in those individuals (females) prone to undervalue their own abilities, and to instill in all students the belief that no one is immune to fire hazards in their lifetime.

REFERENCES

Bandura, A. (1977). Self-efficacy: Towards a unifying theory of behavioral change. *Psychological Review, 84,* 191–215.
Bandura, A. (1982). Self-efficacy mechanisms in human agency. *American Psychologist, 37,* 122–147.

Bandura, A. (1986). *Social foundations of thoughts and action: A social cognitive theory.* Englewood Cliffs, NJ: Prentice-Hall.

Bryan, J. L. (1983). A review of the examination and analysis of the dynamics of human behavior in the fire at the MGM Grand Hotel, Clark County, Nevada, as determined from a selected questionnaire population. *Fire Safety Journal, 5,* 233–240.

Keating, J. P. (1982). The myth of Panic. *Fire Journal, 76,* 57–61.

Paulsen, R. L. (1984). Human behavior and fires: An Introduction. *Fire Technology, 20,* 15–27.

National Safety Council, (1986). *Accident Facts.* Chicago, IL: National Safety Council.

11

SOME ISSUES IN COMPLIANCE WITH ORAL HYGIENE REGIMENS

Jane A. Rankin

Mary B. Harris

The problem of patient noncompliance, a serious issue in the dental and medical literature, was examined within the context of oral hygiene regimens. Subjects were 85 dental professionals and 245 nonprofessional members of the general public. An anonymous questionnaire collected information about demographic data, individuals' oral hygiene practices, dental anxiety, perceptions of oral and physical health, and beliefs about whether their own actions (internality) or the actions of others (externality) were mainly responsible for health.

Professionals reported brushing, flossing, and visiting the dentist more often than nonprofessionals and perceived their physical and dental health as better, as well as scoring lower in dental anxiety than nonprofessionals. Better educated subjects tended to report better health and a lesser perception of control by others, and older subjects reported flossing less often, having poorer physical health, and being lower on internal locus of control. Dental anxiety was negatively correlated with oral hygiene behaviors and perception of dental health. Perceptions of personal control over one's dental health but not over one's general health were weakly positively correlated with frequency of toothbrushing and flossing.

These findings suggest that programs to increase compliance with oral hygiene regimens should consider the characteristics of the subjects, including their level of anxiety, perceptions of internal control, and reasons for noncompliance.

Although good oral hygiene behaviors are known to be important for the maintenance of healthy teeth and gums and for the prevention of future dental problems (Shick, 1981), many dental patients fail to comply with dentists' recommendations concerning toothbrushing and flossing (McCaul

& Glasgow, 1984; Chen & Rubenson, 1982). Not surprisingly, patient noncompliance has been reported as a major problem and source of stress for dentists (Brown, 1981; Corah, O'Shea, & Skeels, 1982). The major purpose of the present study was to examine a number of variables that might be associated with compliance with recommended oral hygiene behaviors, including professional background, demographic variables, dental anxiety, perceptions of control over one's dental health, and perceptions of one's physical and dental health.

DENTAL PROFESSIONALS VS. NONPROFESSIONALS

One objective of this study was to compare oral hygiene behaviors, attitudes about locus of control, frequency of dental visits, perceptions of dental and physical health, and dental anxiety scores in two subpopulations: dental professionals and nonprofessionals.

A study comparing the preventive dental behaviors of hospital employees and their dependents found that physicians were the most prevention-oriented group, followed by nurses, then administrators, technicians, manual workers, and dependents (Antonovsky & Kats, 1970). Nevertheless, Ley (1981) reported that from 12% to 95% of physicians did not comply with the best available medical recommendations. However, based on the assumption that dental professionals are more aware than nonprofessionals of the value of good oral hygiene, it was hypothesized that the oral hygiene scores of dental professionals would be higher than those of nonprofessionals.

Inasmuch as dental professionals are presumably also more aware that self-management is a requirement for effective oral hygiene, it was hypothesized that dental professionals would perceive themselves as more responsible for their dental health than would nonprofessionals. An additional prediction was that dental professionals, owing to their greater knowledge and the desensitizing effects of constant exposure to the dental environment, would score lower on a measure of dental anxiety than would nonprofessionals. It was also expected that dental professionals would visit their own dentist more often, being more aware of the need for such visits than nonprofessionals. As no previous research was found regarding perceptions of dental and physical health with respect to these two subpopulations, no hypotheses about this were formulated.

DEMOGRAPHIC VARIABLES

A second objective of the study was to look at oral hygiene behaviors, frequency of dental visits, perceptions of dental and physical health, and perceptions of control in the general nonprofessional population in respect to four demographic variables: sex, age, ethnicity, and education. Information about the role of demographic variables in patient compliance is inconclusive. In general, the prevailing attitude is that demographic variables do not play an important role in patient compliance (Dunbar & Agras, 1980) and that where a relationship between a demographic variable and patient compliance has been demonstrated, a confounding variable is often found to be responsible. Nevertheless, it seems reasonable to make some predictions.

Oral hygiene. Since Chen and Rubinson (1982) found that wives were more likely than their husbands to floss and brush their teeth regularly, it was hypothesized that the toothbrushing and flossing scores of females would be higher than those of males. Whereas it has been suggested that older people are less interested than younger people in disease prevention (Hurtado, Greenlick, & Columbo, 1973; Jonas, 1971) and that younger and middle-aged individuals use preventive services more often than do older people (Rosenstock & Kirscht, 1979), it was further hypothesized that the toothbrushing and flossing scores of younger and middle-aged individuals would be higher than those of their older counterparts.

There appears to be a positive relationship of level of education with compliance to physicians' recommendations (Kirscht & Rosenstock, 1979) and also with continuing in treatment for chronic conditions (Tagliacozzo & Ima, 1970). Based on this information and on the assumption that better educated people would be more aware of the importance of good oral hygiene practices, it was hypothesized that there would be a positive relationship between level of education and brushing and flossing scores. Because of limited information no prediction were made about the relationship of ethnic background to oral hygiene behaviors.

Frequency of dental visits. Hurtado et al. (1973) found that men were more likely to break medical appointments than were women; Rosenstock and Kirscht (1979) stated that more women than men visit the dentist. Based on this information it was hypothesized that female subjects would have higher dental visit scores than would male subjects. Moreover, since Hurtado et al. (1973) found that failure to keep medical appointments was more common in younger people, it was tentatively hypothesized that there would be a positive relationship between frequency of dental visits and age, while recognizing that factors such as the use of dentures might moderate this relationship.

Some research has found that whites visit physicians and dentists more regularly and are hospitalized more frequently than are nonwhites (Ley,

1981). Based upon this information, it was hypothesized that Anglos would visit the dentist more frequently than would subjects from other ethnic populations. Higher levels of education have also been linked to higher utilization of preventive services (Kirscht & Rosenstock, 1979). Therefore, it was predicted that subjects with higher levels of education would visit the dentist more frequently than would subjects with lower levels of education.

Perceptions of control and health. Although it seems reasonable that ethnic background, age, and gender might be related to perception of control and health, no specific predictions were made. However, based on the assumption that better educated people possess more skills and resources for controlling their own environment, it was expected that subjects who were better educated would perceive themselves as both healthier and as having greater control over their health.

DENTAL ANXIETY

A third objective of the study was to look at the relationship of oral hygiene behaviors to individuals' perceived levels of dental anxiety as measured by scores on the Corah Dental Anxiety Scale (DAS) (Corah, 1969). If dental anxiety motivates people to maintain good oral hygiene habits, one would expect a positive association between DAS scores and brushing scores and between DAS scores and flossing scores; on the other hand, individuals with poor hygiene habits might have more extensive needs for dental care and therefore more anxiety, leading to a negative correlation between the two variables.

PERCEPTIONS OF CONTROL

A final objective of the study was to see whether or not oral hygiene behaviors and other variables were related to perceptions of control over one's dental health. Health locus of control refers to whether individuals feel that their own activities (internal locus of control) are the most important influence on health or illness. It was measured in two ways: by the Multidimensional Health Locus of Control Scale developed by Wallston, Wallston, and DeVellis (1978) and by an author-constructed Dental Locus of Control scale, designed to be more relevant to issues of dentistry. Although two studies had failed to find a significant relationship between perceived control and oral hygiene behaviors (Carnahan, 1980; Harris et al., 1987), a number of theorists have discussed the importance of self-perception of responsibility in affecting health related and even dental behaviors (Davidson, 1982; McCaul & Glasgow, 1984). Accordingly it was predicted that perceived control over one's dental health, as measured by both scales, would be positively related to frequency of flossing and brushing.

METHOD

Subjects

The subjects were 330 individuals who filled out Dental Attitude Questionnaires. These subjects were divided into two groups, depending on whether they only received dental services (patients) or also provided them (dental professionals). There were 85 dental professionals: 26 dentists, 21 hygienists, and 38 students in a university training program for dental assistants and hygienists. This professional group consisted of 26 males and 59 females ranging in age from 20 to 53 years with a median age of 28. Of the 81 dental professionals reporting ethnicity, 9 were Hispanic, 1 was an American Indian, 2 were Black, and 69 were Anglo. Level of education was reported by 82 subjects. Of those reporting, 66% had graduated from or were presently in college, 2% had masters degrees, and 32% had professional dental degrees.

The nonprofessional group consisted of 245 subjects ranging in age from 15 to 81 years with a median age of 33. There were 76 males and 167 females, and 2 subjects whose sex was not reported. Of the 229 who reported ethnicity, 57 were Hispanic, 8 were American Indian, 4 were Black, and 160 were Anglo. Level of education was reported by 236 subjects: 36% reported high school or less education, 52% had graduated from or attended college, 10% had masters degrees, and 1% had completed a Ph.D. or professional degree.

Instrument

The Dental Attitude Questionnaire (DAQ) was an anonymous survey form that requested demograhic data, information about individuals' oral hygiene habits and dental anxiety, perceptions of their dental and physical health, and beliefs about the influence of internal and external forces on their health. The questionnaire included three scales: the Corah Dental Anxiety scale (DAS) (Corah, 1969), the Multidimensional Health Locus of Control scale (MHLC) (Wallston, Wallston, & DeVellis, 1978), and a Dental Control scale (DC) devised by the researchers.

The DAS is a four-item self-report scale widely used in dental research and clinical practice to assess anticipatory anxiety. Each item is scored on a 5-point scale that ranges from 1 = relaxed to 5 = great anxiety.

The purpose of the MHLC scale is to determine whether individuals feel that their general health is more influenced by their own actions or by external factors. Two of the MHLC scales were used in this study: the Internal Health Locus of Control (IHLC) scale and the Powerful Others Health Locus of Control (PHLC) scale. The IHLC scale consists of six questions related to internal locus of control; the PHLC scale consists of six questions related to external locus of control by powerful others such as health professionals. All questions are scored on a 6-point scale that ranges from 1 = strongly disagree to 6 = strongly agree. Thus, the maximum possible total score for each scale is 36; the minimum possible total score is 6.

The DC scale consists of three questions designed to assess subjects' beliefs about whether they control their own dental health. Each of these questions is also scored on a 6-point scale that ranges from 1 = strongly disagree to 6 = strongly agree. The maximum possible total score is 18; the minimum possible total score is 3.

Oral hygiene habits were scored in the following manner. Toothbrushing behaviors were scored on a 5-point scale where 1 = not at all, 2 = once a day, 3 = twice a day, 4 = three times a day, and 5 = more than three times. Flossing behaviors were scored on a 4-point scale where 1 = not at all, 2 = once a day, 3 = twice, and 4 = more than twice. Frequency of dental visits was scored as follows: 1 = never, 2 = only when teeth hurt, 3 = about every two years, 4 = about once a year, and 5 = at least twice a year. Subjects' perceptions of their dental and physical health were both scored as follows: 1 = poor, 2 = fair, 3 = good, and 4 = excellent.

Procedure

The questionnaires were given out at several locations (a dental society meeting, a dental hygiene society meeting, dental offices, a university campus, and a health fair) within a midsize southwestern community, and at a marathon race outside of the city.

Participation in this research project was voluntary. Individuals were asked to read the cover letter explaining the study and to examine the questionnaire before deciding to participate. They were told to leave blank any questions that they did not wish to answer. Those who chose to participate filled out the questionnaire on the spot. Completed questionnaires were then placed in an envelope to be returned to the researchers.

RESULTS

Data for ethnicity and education were categorized in the following ways to facilitate analysis. Analyses of variance were performed comparing only two (Hispanic and Anglo) of the ethnic groups due to the small number of subjects in the other groups. Educational levels for the dental professionals and nonprofessionals were categorized slightly differently because it was necessary to distinguish between postgraduate degrees in the professional group. There are four educational levels for dental professionals: grade through high school, college, masters degree, and PhD or professional degree; but only three educational levels for the nonprofessional general population: grade through high school, college, and postgraduate work.

Dental Professionals vs Nonprofessionals

A multivariate analysis of variance on the difference between dental professionals and nonprofessionals for the variables of toothbrushing, flossing, dental control, internal locus of control, control by professional others, frequency of dental visits, perceptions of dental and physical health, and dental anxiety produced a maximized F ratio of 185.254, yielding a multivariate $F (9,280) = 19.874, p <.001$. The optimal linear combination yielding this F was essentially the sum of the Z scores of all the variables except IHLC, PHLC, and perceptions of physical health. Univariate analyses of variance revealed significant differences between the responses of dental professionals and nonprofessionals in all areas examined as shown in Table 1. Professionals were significantly higher on dental control and internal locus of control but lower on control by powerful others than were nonprofessionals.

An analysis of toothbrushing scores revealed that none of the professionals reported brushing less than twice a day, 37% brushed twice a day, 44% brushed three times a day, and 20% brushed more than three times daily, while 1% of the 235 nonprofessionals reporting did not brush daily, 22% brushed only once, 50% brushed twice a day, 21% brushed three times, and 7% brushed more than three times. An analysis of flossing scores showed that only 10% of the 82 dental professionals reporting did not floss daily, 76% flossed once a day, and 15% flossed twice a day; whereas 53% of the 235 nonprofessionals reporting did not floss daily, 37% flossed once a day, 6% flossed twice a day, and 4% flossed more than twice.

Of the 81 dental professionals reporting their frequency of dental visits, all visited the dentist regularly. Five percent visited the dentist about every two years, 32% about once a year, and 63% at least twice a year; whereas of the

TABLE 1
Dental Professionals vs. Nonprofessionals: A Comparison
of Responses

Variable	X̄ Professionals	X̄ Nonprofessionals	df	F
Toothbrushing	3.83	3.11	1,315	45.91***
Flossing	2.05	1.61	1,315	22.26***
DC score	16.59	14.06	1,318	60.05***
IHLC score	28.73	27.47	1,315	4.34*
PHLC score	15.11	17.09	1,314	7.22**
Frequency of dental visits	4.58	3.87	1,316	28.09***
Perception of dental health	3.66	2.76	1,316	90.75***
Perception of physical health	3.54	3.17	1,317	19.30***
DAS score	6.09	8.98	1,326	44.67***

* $p<.05$
** $p<.01$
*** $p<.001$

237 nonprofessionals reporting on their dental visits, 3% never visited the dentist, 14% said that they visited the dentist only when their teeth hurt, 17% about every two years, 27% about once a year, and 39% at least twice a year.

Perception of oral health was reported by 82 dental professionals: 2% described their oral health as fair, 29% called it good, and 68% said it was excellent. Perception of oral health was reported by 236 nonprofessionals. It was described as poor by 5%, as fair by 31%, as good by 46%, and as excellent by 17%.

Perception of physical health was reported by 82 dental professionals; 46% described their physical health as good, and 54% called it excellent. Perception of physical health was reported by 237 nonprofessionals; 0.4% described their physical health as poor, 15% said it was fair, 51% called it good, and 33% described it as excellent. As predicted, the dental professionals had lower levels of dental anxiety than the nonprofessionals.

Reasons for not brushing and flossing. Table 2 shows how dental professionals and nonprofessionals responded to questions asking why they did not brush or floss as often as recommended. The responses of pro-

TABLE 2
Reasons for Not Brushing or Flossing as Often as Recommended

Reasons	Toothbrushing		Flossing	
	Number of professional responses	Number of nonprofessional responses	Number of nonprofessional responses	Number of nonprofessional responses
Too lazy	8	70	10	65
Forget	7	55	13	54
Not enough time	10	36	11	40
Interferes with activities	6	22	2	15
Don't think necessary	4	19	5	26
Too tired	4	21	8	15
Other reasons	2	17	2	26

fessionals and nonprofessionals were not significantly different with respect to any of the reasons given for not brushing or flossing.

Under other reasons for not brushing, "toothbrush not available" was the reason given most often. Under other reasons for not flossing, "don't like to floss—find it difficult or painful" was the most frequent reason followed by "just don't have the habit."

DEMOGRAPHIC VARIABLES IN THE NONPROFESSIONAL POPULATION

Oral hygiene and frequency of dental visits. Toothbrushing scores did not appear to be significantly related to sex, age, ethnicity, or education. Flossing scores were not significantly related to sex, ethnicity, or education, but were significantly and positively correlated with age, $r(227) = .20, p < .01$. There were no significant relationships between frequency of dental visits and any of the demographic variables.

Perceptions of oral and physical health. There was no significant relationship between subjects' perceptions of their oral health and sex, age, or ethnicity. However, an analysis of variance revealed a significant relationship between subjects' perceptions of their oral health and level of education, $F(2,225) = 4.76, p < .01$.

A post hoc Scheffe' comparison showed that subjects who had a college or postgraduate education, combined $X = 2.85$, perceived their oral health to be better than subjects who had not attended college, $X = 2.54$, $F(1,225) = 6.21$, $p<.05$. Physical health was perceived as significantly better by men, $X = 3.36$, than by women, $X = 3.08$, $F(1,233) = 8.90$, $p<.01$, and a significant low negative correlation was found between perceptions of physical health and age, $r(229) = -.19$, $p<.01$. An analysis of variance revealed that perception of physical health was also significantly related to education, $F(2,226) = 7.29$, $p<.001$. Post hoc Scheffe' comparisons showed that subjects with a college or postgraduate education combined, $X = 3.39$, perceived their physical health to be better than did subjects who had not attended college, $X = 3.00$, $F(1,226) = 17.52$, $p<.01$. There was no significant relationship between perception of physical health and ethnicity. However, perceptions of physical and dental health were significantly positively correlated, $r(234) = .28$, $p<.001$.

DC, IHLC, and PHLC. DC scores were not significantly related to any of the four demographic variables. IHLC scores were not significantly related to sex, ethnicity, or education; but there was a significant negative low correlation between IHLC scores and age, $r(227) = -.13$, $p<.05$. PHLC scores were not significantly related to sex or age; however, an analysis of variance revealed a significant relationship between PHLC scores and ethnicity, $F(1,203) = 7.22$, $p<.01$. The mean scores of Hispanics, $X = 18.88$ were higher than the mean scores of Anglos, $X = 16.27$. There was also a significant relationship between PHLC scores and education, $F(2,221) = 13.07$, $p<.001$. Post hoc Scheffe' comparisons showed that the PHLC scores of subjects who had not attended college $X = 19.68$, were significantly higher than the scores of those with college educations, $X = 15.97$, $F(1,221) = 19.06$, $p<.01$, and than the scores of those with postgraduate educations, $X = 14.23$, $F(1,221) = 16.95$, $p<.01$.

DENTAL ANXIETY

The Pearson product-moment correlations between DAS scores, and toothbrushing, flossing, frequency of dental visits, and perception of dental health were significant and negative for all subjects combined, as shown in Table 3. Only correlations between DAS scores and flossing, dental visit frequency, and perception of dental health were significant and negative for nonprofessional subjects. DAS scores were not significantly correlated with any of the other variables for dental professionals. Nor were they significantly associated with IHLC scores, PHLC scores, or DC scores for professionals or

TABLE 3
Pearson Product-Moment Correlations of Selected Variables with Dental Anxiety Scale Scores

Correlation with DAS Scores	All Subjects[a]	Dental Professionals	Nonprofessionals
Toothbrushing	−.15(313)**	−.00(80)	−.04(231)
Flossing	−.21(313)***	−.13(80)	−.13(231)*
Dental visit frequency	−.32(314)***	.06(79)	−.27(233)***
Perception of dental health	−.27(314)***	−.14(80)	−.14(232)*
DC	−.18(316)***	−.16(83)	−.04(231)
IHLC	−.06(313)	.01(81)	−.03(230)
PHLC	−.06(312)	.02(82)	.01(228)

* $p<.05$
** $p<.01$
*** $p<.001$
[a]—Degrees of freedom are in parentheses.

nonprofessionals considered separately. However, there was a significant but low negative correlation between DAS scores and DC scores for all subjects combined.

LOCUS OF CONTROL SCALES

The mean scores for the subjects in our sample on the IHLC scale ($X = 27.80$) were somewhat higher than the mean scores reported for the IHLC by Wallston and Wallston (1981) which ranged from 25.55 to 27.38 for various samples. Similarly, our subjects had somewhat lower scores on the PHLC scale ($X = 16.57$) than the sample means of 17.87 to 19.16 reported by Wallston and Wallston (1981). Our subjects scored significantly higher on the IHLC scale than Wallston and Wallston's healthy adults and college students and significantly lower on the PHLC scale than these groups as well as their subjects engaging in preventive health care behaviors, lowest $t(316) = 4.19$, $p<.001$. Similar results were found for our subgroups of dental professionals and nonprofessionals considered separately. All of this suggests that our subjects may have a greater sense of internal control and a lesser sense of being controlled by powerful others than the normative sample.

Toothbrushing scores for the entire sample were not significantly related to IHLC scores or PHLC scores, but the relationship between brushing scores and DC scores for all subjects was significant and positive although low, $r(307) = .15$, $p<.01$. Nor was there any significant relationship between flossing scores for the entire sample and IHLC scores or PHLC scores.

However, the relationship between flossing scores for all subjects and DC scores was significant and positive but also low, $r(306) = .11, p<.05$. Neither IHLC, PHLC, nor DC scores were significantly correlated with brushing or flossing scores for dental professionals or nonprofessionals considered separately.

MULTIPLE REGRESSION ANALYSES

The relationships of professional status, dental control, internal locus of control, control by powerful others, frequency of dental visits, perception of dental and physical health, and dental anxiety scores to toothbrushing and to flossing were examined via unique multiple regression analyses. The multiple R for frequency of toothbrushing was .457, accounting for 21% of the variance, $F (8,282) = 9.31$, p <.01. Three predictor variables contributed significantly to the regression equation for toothbrushing: professional status, $F (1,282) = 12.59, p <.01$, accounting for 4% of the variance (based on the squared part correlation); perception of dental health, $F (1,282) = 11.72, p <.01$, accounting for 3% of the variance; and frequency of dental visits, $F (1,282) = 4.50, p <.05$, accounting for 1% of the variance. The multiple R for flossing was .357, accounting for 13% of the variance, $F (8,281) = 5.12, p <.01$. The only variable that contributed significantly to the regression equation for flossing was professional status, $F (1,281) = 5.78, p <.05$.

DISCUSSION

The findings of this study are limited by the sampling procedures used and thus cannot necessarily be generalized to all dental patients or professionals. Nevertheless, the fact that subjects did represent a variety of backgrounds with respect to age, ethnicity, and gender suggests that the results may have some general implications.

Dental Professionals vs Nonprofessionals

The professionals who responded to the questionnaire were more inclined toward internality, less inclined toward externality, and reported more brushing and flossing activity. Moreover, dental professionals experienced less anxiety about dental treatment, visited their dentists more frequently, and perceived their oral health as well as their physical health to be better than did nonprofessionals. All of this indicated that the attitudes, beliefs, and behaviors of dental professionals reflect a greater concern than those of nonprofessionals with issues related to prevention and maintenance.

The question is: What can be done to help the nonprofessional general public become more like the dental professional population in these respects? Past research has shown that self-management and self-efficacy are both linked to internality (Lefcourt, 1982) and also to compliance (Davidson, 1982; Lefcourt, 1982). If dental patients could be taught the skills of self-management as well as the correct procedures for brushing and flossing, they might increase their level of perceived control over their oral health and decrease their level of dental anxiety to approach the scores of dental professionals. These changes in self-perception might then serve as mediators to increase the level of compliance with oral hygiene regimens.

Reasons For Noncompliance

Dental professionals and nonprofessionals were most alike when stating reasons for not complying with recommended oral hygiene procedures. Although the order varied for professionals and nonprofessionals as well as for toothbrushing and flossing behaviors, the three most frequently reported reasons were: laziness, forgetting, and not enough time. It was not surprising that some members of the nonprofessional group did not think it necessary to brush or floss as often as recommended, but it was surprising to find that there were also members of the dental professionals group who felt this way. These findings suggest that, in some cases, reasons for not complying may be as compelling as reasons for complying and, therefore, should always be considered when designing programs to increase compliance.

Demographic Variables

In general, the demographic variables of sex, age, education, and ethnicity were not significantly associated with oral hygiene behaviors, with the exception of the slight tendency for older subjects to floss less often.

The fact that subjects who were better educated and who were Anglos perceived themselves as less controlled by others, and that younger subjects perceived themselves as more internally controlled than older ones may reflect the actual realities of peoples' situations and resources. The differences between dental professionals and their nonprofessional counterparts are consistent with this interpretation.

Although a significant and positive correlation was found between subjects' perceptions of their oral and physical health, only education was significantly related to both the perception of oral health and the perception of physical health. Subjects who had attended college perceived both their oral and physical health to be better than those who reported having less education. Perception of oral health was not significantly related to any of the other three demographic variables, nor was perception of physical health significantly related to ethnicity. However, it was found that males perceived their physical health to be significantly better than did females and that there was a significant decline in how subjects rated their perceived state of health as they grew older.

As mentioned earlier, younger subjects tended to see themselves as more internally controlled, with Hispanics and less educated subjects perceiving powerful others as exerting relatively more control over their health. However, in general, demographic variables had little or no influence on compliance or variables associated with it, which is congruent with the findings in the medical literature (Dunbar & Agras, 1980; Rosenstock & Kirscht, 1979).

Dental Anxiety

The results of this study suggest that dental anxiety does not serve as a motivator for oral hygiene behavior, but rather that people with better oral hygiene practices have less anxiety when in the dentists' chair. The causal pathways for this relationship are unclear, but the low negative correlation between dental anxiety and perceived control over one's dental health suggests the possibility that having a sense of control may reduce anxiety, which in turn may lead to more frequent visits to the dentist. Whether more frequent brushing and flossing decrease anxiety directly or whether a sense of control affects anxiety and oral hygiene behaviors independently is a matter to be determined by future research.

Health Locus of Control

The results of this study provide only weak evidence that locus of control is a factor influencing oral hygiene behaviors. Neither the IHLC scale nor the PHLC scale was significantly associated with oral hygiene behaviors in our sample, nor in the subjects studied by Carnahan (1980). On the other hand, a brief scale designed to measure specific beliefs about one's control over dental health did show positive correlations between internality and brushing and flossing for the entire sample. Just as research on locus of control has shifted from generalized notions of control to studying perceptions of control in particular areas such as health, it may be that an even narrower focus, specifically on oral health, might lead to greater precision in predicting oral hygiene behaviors. Further development and modification of the DC scale to increase its reliability and validity would be a necessary next step.

CONCLUSIONS

The results of multiple regression analyses suggested that the most powerful predictor of oral hygiene behaviors was professional status, although a more positive perception of one's dental health and more frequent visits to the dentist were also associated with more frequent toothbrushing.

Although the findings were inconclusive regarding the relationship of internality and oral hygiene behaviors, enough evidence of a positive relationship was forthcoming to recommend the development of programs to instruct the general public in ways to utilize the components (self-management and self-efficacy) of internality to increase their oral hygiene activities (Rankin & Harris, 1987). It is also suggested that programs designed to increase compliance should recognize the importance of reasons for noncompliance as well as the influence that some demographic variables may have on factors affecting compliance. Such programs may have an effect not only on brushing and flossing but also on dental anxiety, which in turn may influence frequency of visiting the dentist and one's state of dental health. Not surprisingly, dental professionals appear to have less dental anxiety, better oral hygiene habits, and a greater sense of control over their health than nonprofessionals. One outcome of a good self-management program might be to have nonprofessional dental patients become more like dental professionals in these respects.

REFERENCES

Antonovsky, A., & Kats, R. (1970). The model dental patient: An empirical study of preventive health behavior. *Social Science and Medicine, 4,* 367–380.

Brown, J. C. (1981). Patient noncompliance: A neglected topic in dentistry. *Journal of the American Dental Association, 103*(4), 567–569.

Carnahan, T. M. (1980). The development and validation of the multi-dimensional dental locus of control scales (Doctoral dissertation, State University of New York). *Dissertation Abstracts International, 41*A, 591.

Chen, M., & Rubinson, L. (1982). Preventive dental behavior in families: A national survey. *Journal of the American Dental Association, 105*(7), 43–46.

Corah, N. L. (1969). Development of a dental anxiety scale. *Journal of Dental Research, 48,* 596.

Corah, N. L., O'Shea, R. M., & Skeels, D. K. (1982). Dentists' perceptions of problem behaviors in patients. *Journal of the American Dental Association, 104*(6), 829–833.

Davidson, P. O. (1982). Issues in patient compliance. In T. Millon, C. Green, & R. Menger (Eds.), *Handbook of clinical health psychology* (pp. 417–434). New York: Plenum.

Dunbar, J. M., & Agras, W. S. (1980). Compliance with medical instructions. In J. M. Ferguson & C. B. Taylor (Eds.), *The comprehensive handbook of behavioral medicine* (Vol. 3, pp. 115–145). New York: Medical and Scientific Books.

Harris, M. B., Jackman, L. E., Tonigan, J. S., Dempsey, T. J., Holburn, S., Sawey, J., & Herlan, M. (1987). Knowledge, locus of control and dental care behaviors. *Journal of Compliance in Health Care, 2*(2), 155–165.

Hurtado, A. V., Greenlick, M. R., & Colombo, T. J. (1973). Determinants of medical care utilization: Failure to keep appointments. *Medical Care, 11,* 189–198.

Jonas, S. (1971). Appointment breaking in a general medical clinic. *Medical Care, 9,* 82–88.

Kirscht, J. F., & Rosenstock, I. M. (1979). Patients' problems in following health recommendations of health experts. In G. Stine, F. Cohen, & N. Adler (Eds.), *Health psychology: A handbook* (pp. 189–215). San Francisco: Jossey-Bass.

Lefcourt, H. M. (1982). *Locus of control* (2nd ed.). Hillsdale, NJ: Lawrence Erlbaum.

Ley, P. (1981). Professional noncompliance: A neglected problem. *British Journal of Clinical Psychology, 20*(3), 151–154.

Ley, P. (1982). Satisfaction, compliance, and communication. *British Journal of Clinical Psychology, 21*(4), 241–254.

McCaul, K. D., & Glasgow, R. E. (1984). Health psychology: Adherence to preventive dental regimens. *Contemporary Social Psychology, 10*(3), 45–48.

Rankin, J. A., & Harris, M. B. (1987). Using self-control instructions to change oral hygiene habits: A pilot study. *New Mexico Dental Journal, 38*(1), 7–15.

Rosenstock, I. M., & Kirscht, J. P. (1979). Why people seek health care. In G. Stine, F. Cohen, & N. Adler (Eds.), *Health psychology: A handbook* (pp. 161–188). San Francisco: Jossey-Bass.

Shick, R. A. (1981). Maintenance phase of periodontal therapy. *Journal of Periodontology, 52*(9), 576–583.

Tagliacozzo, D., & Ima, K. (1970). Knowledge of illness as a mediator of patient behavior. *Journal of Chronic Diseases, 22,* 765–775.

Wallston, K. A., & Wallston, B. S. (1981). Health locus of control scales. In H. Lefcourt (Ed.), *Research with the locus of control construct* (1, 189–243). New York: Academic Press.

Wallston, K. A., Wallston, B. S., & De Vellis, R. (1978). Development of the multidimensional health locus of control (MHLC) scales. *Health Education Monographs, 6,* 160–170.

The authors wish to express their appreciation to the Albuquerque District Dental Society and the Albuquerque District Dental Hygiene Society for their assistance in distributing the Dental Attitude Questionnaires.

12

GERONTOLOGICAL HEALTH EDUCATION RESEARCH: ISSUES AND RECOMMENDATIONS

Suzanne Laidlaw Feldman

The fastest growing segment of the population in the United States is the age group over 65. The health education needs for this population are diverse ranging from driver education to patient education concerning incontinence. Yet very few health education programs are designed for the elderly. Reasons for the lack of health education programs are discussed. The influence of the medical model in defining health of the elderly is offered as a primary reason for the lack of health education for the elderly. Society's negative view of aging is also discussed. In part II of this paper, new models are proposed for gerontological health education. The life span perspective of aging is combined with the wellness perspective of health. Comprehensive gerontological health education is defined. The ecological aspects of health education programs are discussed. In Part III, cognitive and family life span developmental theories are discussed and applied to gerontological health education. Methodological issues, such as cohort effects and population derived definitions of health, are discussed. The article is concluded by proposing that health educators need to play a more dominate role in gerontology.

When Mrs. Janice Brown went for her yearly physical, she had many concerns that she wanted to discuss with her physician. She was worried that her arthritis, though mild, was affecting her intimacy with her husband. Sexual intercourse was painful and not as satisfying as it had been. However, she did not feel comfortable discussing these intimate problems with her physician. She wondered what he would think of a 75-year-old woman concerned about this matter. She left the interview without mentioning her concerns. Her physician, in turn, failed to ask her about her emotional and sexual well-being. His focus was on the medical aspects of her arthritis.

This vignette is just one of many that illustrates the need for health education for older adults and gatekeepers. The purpose of this paper is to provide a new framework for health education research and programs for older adults.

In the United States, the fastest growing segment of the population is the age group 65 and older. In 1980, there were 25.7 million elderly[1] as compared to 16.6 million elderly in 1960 (U.S. Bureau of Census, 1984). Within the elderly population, the greatest change has occurred among those over the age of 85. In 1980, 2.3 million people were over 85 years of age as compared to .9 million people 85 or older in 1960. Though it is unknown what precise effect the AIDS epidemic will have on survivorship into older adulthood, it is expected that the trend of an increase in the elderly population will continue into the 21st century with the aging of the post-World War II baby-boom generation (e.g. Zopf, 1986). Rosenwaike & Dolinsky (1987) predict that life expectancy at ages 65 and 75 will be 20 years and 15 years, respectively, by the year 2000.

The elderly constitute a heterogeneous population. Within population, variability occurs for many demographic characteristics such as income and living arrangements, and along a number of psychological and social dimensions (U.S. Bureau of Census, 1984; Zopf, 1986; Krauss, 1980). There is also diversity for health status and health needs. Consequently, there has been an expanding need for a variety of health education programs and research for older adults. The health education needs range from defensive driving education to patient education concerning incontinence.

However, though there is an increasing need for gerontological health education research, very little research has been conducted. There has been a paucity of experimental or quasi-experimental gerontological health education research. Most of the published studies have been descriptive. Minkler (1984) states that health promotion, which includes health education, is a "foreign concept in relation to the elderly" (p. 77). More studies have been published in 1987 about health education and the elderly than in 1984; however, the amount is limited when compared to other areas in health education. To illustrate this point, it is noted that *Ageline,* which is a bibliographic database on aging, does not include health education journals, such as *Health Education Quarterly* and *Health Education* (American Association of Retired Persons, 1987). In this article many of the cited

---

[1]Elderly is defined as persons aged 65 or older. This age, though arbitrary, is used to be consistent with previous definitions (Zopf, 1986). It is noted that the term elderly sometimes has a pejorative connotation. In this chapter, it is used solely to define a population by chronological age. No other meaning is implied.

research studies were published in gerontological or aging journals and not in health education journals. Most of the articles are not referenced within health education, but in other domains, such as health behavior or patient care research.

In Part I, reasons for the lack of health education research concerning the elderly are discussed. The problems of defining health, aging, and health education for older adults are explored. In part II, new perspectives toward health education for older adults are proposed. The salutogenic model (Antonovsky, 1984) of health is suggested as an alternative to the medical model. Life span developmental perspective is offered as an orientation to aging. Comprehensive gerontological health education is defined and proposed as a useful approach to health education. It is suggested that the ecological perspective be incorporated into the health education paradigm. In Part III, relevant theories and research from life span developmental psychology are presented. Applications to health education are given. Methodological issues are discussed.

PART I

Issues in Defining Health and Aging

How one defines health and aging influences what form health education will take, if any. What does it mean to be a healthy 75-year-old person, or a healthy 90-year-old person? Is it an impossibility to be simultaneously healthy and 90 years old? Many would answer yes to this question. Although many health educators define health from a wellness perspective, this orientation has not been applied to the older adult to the same degree as to younger populations. A traditional medical perspective of health has been maintained. With the medical model, a person is classified according to disease categories. Today, the disease categories have been expanded to include chronic as well as acute diseases. If an individual has symptoms, then the individual is categorized as having a disease or condition, and defined as a patient in need of care. If a person cannot be classified into a disease category, then the individual is considered healthy. Health, therefore, is defined as the absence of disease. Health status is determined by the presence or absence of diseases for a population at a particular place and time (Lilienfield & Lilienfeld, 1980). Therefore, morbidity and mortality rates are derived to index health. Within medicine, the specialty of geriatrics has developed that "deals with the problems and diseases of old age and aging people" (Webster's New Collegiate Dictionary, 1974).

The concept of aging and the concept of disease have been intertwined. To be old has been equated with being diseased. Also, the aging process has been perceived as an inevitable, declining process. For example, many people believe that a consequence of growing old is the development of Alzheimer's disease. Even today, many would agree with Shakespeare when he wrote:

> That ends this strange eventful history, Is second childishness, and mere oblivion, Sans teeth, sans eyes, sans taste, sans every thing.
>
> (Act II, vii, *As You Like It*)

By narrowly defining health and aging in this manner, a perplexing problem arises. According to this perspective, older adults are, by definition, "less healthy" than younger adults because the life expectancy for older adults is less than that of younger adults. Also, morbidity rates for chronic diseases are higher for older adults than younger adults.

Consequently, interventions to improve the health of older adults are designed from a medical orientation. Professionals who have training in the medical professions play a dominate role in determining health programs, services, and research concerning the elderly. Therefore, interventions are designed to alleviate symptoms and provide medical services rather than prevent disease or promote wellness through health education. Regrettably, often the goals of alleviating symptoms and providing minimal medical care are not achieved for the elderly. Health care finance programs, such as Medicare, were designed to fund short-term hospitalizations and not designed for long-term care for chronic conditions (Minkler, 1984). In a recent report (Wolfe, 1988) it was found that basic medical services may not be provided through Medicaid. Medicaid, a joint federal-state program, was designed to fund medical services for poor people, including the poor elderly. It was found that gross inequalities exist between states. For example, in California, rehabilitative therapy is funded, but in Texas, this is not funded at all.

By defining health in this manner, differences in perceived health may exist between older adults and health care providers. Sometimes "symptoms" may be assumed to exist because of an individual's age that, in fact, do not exist. For example, it may be assumed because of a person's age that the individual is forgetful, even though he or she may not be. Conversely, "symptoms" of a disease or side effects of medication may be attributed to aging, not to other causes and, therefore, assumed to be inevitable. As in the case above, symptoms of memory loss may be attributed to aging but, in this case, be due to side effects of medication. Though the "symptom" is correctable, nothing may be done about it. These perceptions of "symptoms" may be held by either the client/patient or the health care provider, or both. Prohaska, Keller, Leventhal, and Leventhal (1987) found that when symptoms were perceived as vague and mild, they were attributed to aging by older adults. Older adults were more likely to delay treatment for the mild symptoms. However, if the symptoms were "severe and acute," older adults were less likely to attribute the symptoms to aging.

In addition, the situation is more complicated. Sometimes symptoms of a disease or condition may vary with age. For example, symptoms of a heart attack may include pain for a younger adult, but no pain for an older adult. Erroneously, people may assume that the disease or condition is not present because it does not fit the typical symptomatology.

Wison and Netting (1987) compared health care providers' (registered nurses, pharmacists, social workers, etc.) perceptions of the health of community-based elderly with the older adults' perceptions of their own health. Among a number of findings, the researchers found incongruence between the elderly's perceptions of health and barriers to service as compared to the health care providers' perceptions. The health care providers perceived the elderly as having more specific health problems than the elderly perceived themselves as having. Also, they perceived the elderly as being hospitalized more than they actually were.

Rakowski, Hickey, and Dengiz (1987) also investigated the agreement in perception of health and treatment between health care providers (physicians, residents, and clinic nurse specialists), and elderly patients at a university clinic. Congruence varied from 29% to 69% for 14 health and treatment questions.

Keyes, Bisno, Richardson, and Mueston (1987) examined the relationship between age and dysfunctioning following colostomy surgery. They expected to find older subjects to be more dysfunctional than younger subjects. They found no greater incidence of depression or dysfunctioning among older patients than among younger patients. Differences in type of coping correlated with age however.

In an ethnographic study of community-living elderly, Mitterness (1987) found that approximately 30% of the elderly residents had urinary incontinence at least once a week. One-third of these elderly persons never mentioned it to their physicians. They didn't believe that there was anything that could be done about the problem. Of those who did mention it to their physicians, 48% of the physicians ignored the "symptom" or minimized it.

Concluding from the cited research, defining health and aging in relation to disease limits the opportunities for health education for older adults and also leads to limited medical care as well. This approach is in opposition to the fact that most older adults are independent, functioning persons (U.S. Bureau of the Census, 1984). This approach is also in opposition to the needs of the frail, institutionalized elderly as well. In addition, this approach does not account for the fact that the majority of older adults define their health as excellent or good, even though a large percentage of older adults have chronic health problems.

Issues In Defining Health Education

According to Green, Kreuter, Deeds, and Partridge (1980), health education is defined as "any combination of learning experiences designed to facilitate voluntary adaptation of behavior conducive to health" (p. 7). The target population for the health education may be the individual whose health is being considered, or the "decision-makers, opinion leaders, and 'gatekeepers'" who have an impact on the individual (Green, 1984, p. 187). Green (1984) considers health education to be a part of health promotion. Health promotion includes not only health education but also nonbehavioral techniques, such as, economic and environmental interventions that improve health. Others, such as Matarazzo (1984), use the term health enhancement or promotion to refer to programs that focus on behaviors that promote wellness and/or are preventive in focus.

As described in the PRECEDE Model (Green et al., 1980) there are three sets of modifible factors that influence health behavior. One set is the *predisposing* variables, such as the beliefs and attitudes of the participants; the second set is the *enabling* variables, such as the skills and barriers present; and the third set are the *reinforcing* variables, such as the supportive "feedback" from others. Therefore, health education research may focus on a variety of processes or variables, including needs assessment, attitude change, or evaluation research.

With the above definition of health education, three issues of importance need to be discussed as they relate to the older adult. The first issue is that of voluntary participation. The second and third issues relate to two fundamental assumptions inherent in this definition. The first assumption is that there is a relationship between health behavior and health status; that is, the assumption that if one changes health behavior, this change will have an effect on health status. The second assumption is that health education interventions or techniques can facilitate changes in health behavior; that is, there are interventions to help the individual change his or her behavior. Much of health education research is aimed at delineating what are effective techniques.

A key component of health education programs is the presence of "voluntary participation" (Green, 1984). According to Green, participants need to take an active role in their education. However, the issue of active, voluntary participation is problematic when considering the elderly. Before it is possible to have participation, there first must be programs available and research conducted. Therefore, funding must be available for such endeavors. As discussed in the previous section, our society has a limited view of aging and health. Stereotyping by the gatekeepers leads to limited availability of programs. The stereotyping is a complex process, as will be illustrated in the cited research (see Braithwaite, Gibson, & Holman, 1985–86).

The gatekeepers may be at the societal, institutional, and/or individual level. Also, individual older adults are gatekeepers themselves as to whether or not they will disclose information to health care providers, or participate in programs. Gatekeepers influence each other synergistically. For example, funding provided by the policymakers influences which research is given priority. The research results and interests of the health educators influence what funding requests are made. What is reported in the popular press is influenced by funding and research priorities. This in turn influences society's attitudes, which is reflected in what the policymakers fund, and so on. In Table 1 a list of gatekeepers of gerontological health education and health promotion is presented. Examples of what gatekeepers control are given.

In a content analysis of published congressional speeches, Luboudrov (1987) found that most congress members used stereotypes when describing the elderly. Interestingly, both negative and positive themes occurred, such as perceiving the elderly to be in poor health, unable to change, or living in institutions; or to be financially well off, make friends easily, and be good listeners. Stereotypes were used by advocates who were promoting funding for the elderly, as well as by those in favor of decreasing funding for the elderly.

What are health educators attitudes and perceptions of older adults? Do health educators provide programs or conduct research with older adults? Traditionally, a significant portion of health education programs have been designed for children and adolescents through school health education programs. Community public health education programs are, as indicated in the name, community wide in scope; therefore, these programs are usually oriented to all members of the community. Consequently, adults are treated as if they are members of a homogenous population. The needs of the subpopulations of adults are not always considered. For example, in a study of patient medication instruction, the patients ranged in age from 35 to 79 years of age (De Tullio, et al., 1986). Consequently, very few studies or

TABLE 1
Examples of Gatekeepers of Gerontological Health Education and Promotion

Gatekeepers	Control
Society:	
Members	Prevailing attitudes
Organizations	Dessemination of information
Policymakers	Advocacy
	Funding
Educators and Researchers:	
Gerontologists	Theories and research
Health educators	Education of health-care providers
Sociologists	Models & projects
Psychologists	
Institutional Personnel:	
Administrators	Programs available
Staff:	Role definitions
Activity Therapists	Attitudes about health and aging
Nurses	Program facilitators or instructors
Direct Care Workers	
Health-Care Providers:	
Physicians	Patient education
Nurses	Pharmocological education
Dentists	Nutrition education
Nutritionists	
Pharmacists	
Social Workers	
Psychologists	
Family Members and Peer Group:	
Spouse	Financial support
Siblings	Social support
Adult Children	Decision-making
Friends	Sources of information and education
Older Adults:	
	Participation
	Decision-making
	Attitude, knowledge, & behavior change

programs are designed specifically for the elderly. In a recent issue of *Health Education Quarterly* that was devoted to asthma and asthma management, Wilson-Pessano et al. (1987) state that there has been little research on the topic of asthma education and adults. There has been even less research on the older adult and asthma. In some cases, older adults are excluded from samples within health education research. For example, though there is much research on health education and AIDS, there is little known about the health needs and health education needs of the older homosexual male. (See special issue of *Health Education Quarterly*, 1986, on AIDS education.)

In research that is published in gerontology journals, in which most participants are older adult subjects, the focus on health is more likely to be from a medical perspective. Health educators do not play a dominant role in the gerontology field. An indication of the lack of participation by health educators is the fact that of 189 Gerontology Fellowships awarded between 1979 to 1984, only one was given to a health educator (Hoffand, Smyer, Wetle, & Walter, 1987). However, one-half to two-thirds of the programs were health or medically related, such as program development, evaluation, and needs assessment. Clearly, these topics are within the domain of health education research.

At the patient-health care provider level there also is a biasing against accessibility of information or responding to the older patient/client. Greene, Hoffman, Charon, and Adelman (1987) analyzed the types of interactions that occurred between physicians and patients. In this study, the medical interviews of five physicians each with four younger patients (45 years and less), and four older patients (65 years and greater) were analyzed according to who initiated concerns, and how the concerns were handled. Physicians were more responsive to younger patients' concerns. The issue as to why physicians responded differently was not investigated.

Ray, McKinney, and Ford (1987) examined the attitudes that clinical psychologists hold toward patients labeled as "older" or "younger." A sample of clinical psychologists responded to mailed questionaires. The clinical psychologists were asked to determine prognoses and placements of clients who were described in vignettes. It was found that prognosis and placement varied with age and type of category. For example, older clients were rated as having a lower prognosis for depression than younger clients. However, no difference was found for alcohol abuse prognosis. The authors did not address the issue of why there were differences in predictions. Perhaps clinical psychologists hold more negative attitudes, or perhaps they perceived older clients as experiencing more barriers to care.

Minkler (1984), in addressing the need for health promotion for the elderly in long-term care facilities, states that the long-term care facility is a "dependency-producing environment" (p. 78). This environment works in opposition to providing health promotion/education; that is, active participation is discouraged. According to Minkler, health promotion needs to be provided to the gatekeepers as well as the residents. Minkler emphasizes that it would not only be ineffective to focus solely on the residents, but more importantly, it would be unethical.

Older adults themselves may not have information, or may not perceive themselves as active participants. As previously mentioned in the Mitterness study (1987), older adults may lack knowledge about the control of incontinence. Lasoski and Thelen (1987) assessed attitudes and knowledge about mental health services among the elderly. They found that "lack of knowledge by the elderly concerning outpatient health services . . . is the most highly rated reason for low usage . . ." (Lasoski & Thelen, 1987, p. 292) Kushman and Freeman (1986) also found differences in awareness and knowledge of services among older adults. For example, older males were less knowledgeable than older females about homemaker services, such as Meals-on-Wheels.

Accessibility to health education by older ethnic minority adults may be even more limited than for older adults in general. Additional barriers, such as language, food practices, or cultural customs may limit access to health education. Koh and Bell (1987) found that most older Korean adults do not utilize typical Western health services, but instead visit Korean medical or herbal doctors. In a nonrandom sample of Hispanic older adults, aged 55 and older, Bastida (1987) found differences between males and females about what, how, and to whom one discusses heterosexual relationships. These attitudes and preferences may influence whether sexual information (or education) is sought, and from whom it is sought.

The second issue, the relationship between changes in health behavior with a correlated change in health status, is crucial to determining whether or not a program is effective. Though the success of a particular program is evaluated by changes in health knowledge, attitudes, or behavior, the ultimate success is dependent upon the linkage between health behavior and health status. Therefore, an effective program not only leads to changes in health behavior, but also (however limited this might be) leads to increases in life expectancy. By defining success in this manner, older adults are sometimes excluded from health education programs because it is not perceived as cost effective to increase life expectancy at the upper age level. Minkler (1984) refers to this as the youth bias of health promotion. Why should one invest energy and time with an older population—it is too little, too late. Being old and near death is precisely what one is trying to avoid, so goes the argument.

Ironically, this approach can lead to contradictory results. For example, though the mortality rate due to stroke has decreased, the morbidity rate has increased (Baum, 1987). The need for health services and education may have increased.

The third issue, that effective health education techniques can facilitate health behavior change, has been assumed not to be applicable to older adult populations. Green et al. (1980) state that the "earlier the [health education] intervention occurs in growth and development of the subjects, the greater the probability of change (p. 60). Older adults are perceived as set in their ways, unchangeable, and unable to learn. This is a strong bias held by the gatekeepers. Interestingly, adult developmental psychology literature indicates that change and learning are possible, and in fact do occur throughout adulthood. Factors such as level of education, activity in adulthood, health status, and occupation are better predictors of memory and learning than is chronological age.

Consequently, there is a need for a new perspective for health education for older adults. In Part II, comprehensive gerontological health education is proposed as an alternative.

PART II

New Approaches to Health and Aging

According to Kuhn (1970), "a paradigm is what the members of a scientific community share" (p. 176). A paradigm is a "disciplinary matrix," that is, the "shared commitments to belief" and "values" held by the community (Kuhn, 1970, p. 188). Paradigms determine theories and how research hypotheses will be investigated; they also determine the interpretation of research results. More fundamentally, however, a paradigm determines if a research hypothesis will be considered for investigation. The discipline matrix or paradigm for a scientific community is the framework that the members utilize when considering what is legitimate and within the acceptable domain of the community.

Wellness Perspective

What is the health education paradigm? Green (1984) states that health education has three main traditional orientations, that is, school health education, community health education, and patient health education. Education and, more specifically, changes in health knowledge, were considered the primary goal of health education. Historically, priorities were the prevention of contagious diseases, hygiene, and decreasing "immoral behavior" such as drinking alcohol (Kime, Schlaadt, and Tritsch, 1977).

Today, health education is in a state of flux and in a "preparadigmatic state", or in "paradigmatic shift", depending upon your viewpoint. There is movement from a focus on disease prevention to a wellness orientation. Antonovsky's (1984) salutogenic model is an illustration of this change. There has been a shift from solely focusing on knowledge change to including changes in health skills and behavior. Also, a shift has occurred from considering health education to the broader perspective of health promotion (Green, 1984).

This shift has been very limited for health education for the elderly as was previously discussed. Since the medical-disease model is dominant, the focus on wellness and health promotion for older adults has been quite limited. It is argued by the present author that gerontological health education falls within the domain of health education; the paradigm of gerontological health education is not the same perspective as found in geriatrics. How one best promotes wellness for ninety-year-old persons is a legitimate research question for investigation by health educators. Consequently, there needs to be a change or expansion in considering what constitutes wellness, adult development, and health education.

To highlight this point, consider the issue of time management for reducing risk and developing a health enhancing life-style (Everly, 1985). According to Everly, an individual needs to learn how to "manage oneself" in relation to time, both in terms of risk reduction and also in terms of providing time to change life-style. Time management education can be thought of as a prerequisite to other health education programs. The tendency is to perceive time management education as a need for younger working adults only. However, results from a study conducted by Quinn and Keznikoff (1985) would lead one to question this assumption. Quinn and Keznikoff (1985) found that death anxiety correlated positively with "inefficient use of time, lack of direction in lives, and a sense of time pressure" (p. 197). In this study, the sample of subjects consisted of members of a senior citizen center. The authors relate their findings to suicide prevention. Time management education may also be a useful intervention for the older adult population. Moreover, it could be argued that there may be a greater need for time management education for the older adult than the younger adult. The older adult needs to adapt to the change from being work oriented to being leisure oriented or nonwork oriented.

Kiyak's (1984) research and programs on oral health promotion for the elderly is an excellent example of how the shift in perspective from disease to wellness can occur for the elderly. Kiyak cogently argues that edentulous older adults need preventive dental intervention, not only to prevent diseases of the mouth due to improper fitting dentures but also because of the impact the health of the mouth can have on one's speech, eating behavior (and therefore, nutritional status), esthetics, and total well-being. Kiyak defines and assesses preventive dentistry differently for older adults than for younger populations. For children or younger adults, preventive dentistry may focus on the prevention of caries and gum diseases. For the older adult, the focus is on the prevention of further disease, and/or the improvement in chewing behavior or speech with the use of properly fitting dentures.

Another example of this shift is the Staying Healthy After Fifty (SHAF) program, which is a health education program for older adults (Kane-Williams, 1987). This program is an expansion of the Self-Care for Senior Citizens (SCSC) program (Nelson et al, 1984). Throughout the course, responsibility for personal health is emphasized. The SHAF program consists of 22 hours of class time in which participants acquire knowledge and skills about health practices and community services. In this program, there are sessions on medical issues such as, blood pressure. Also, there are sessions on life-style, such as, emotional well-being, in which participants learn progressive relaxation techniques. Active learning techniques are employed. In the original program (1984), improvement was found for health knowledge, skill performance, and confidence in performing skills. No differences were found between the control group and the intervention group on measures of medical care utilization, or health status.

The previously cited programs illustrate the application of the wellness perspective to health education for older adults. It is suggested that the salutogenic model developed by Antonovsky (1979, 1984) is an appropriate model of health for gerontological health education. Antonovsky theorizes that the pathogenetic model of disease be expanded to include a focus on health, well-being, and adaptation. With this expansion in viewpoint, rather than thinking of an individual as being classified according to disease categories, an individual is placed along a continuum between total health and total illness. According to Antonovsky (1984), one examines how the individual copes, and "what facilitates one's becoming healthier" (p. 117).

Combining this perspective with the biopsychosocial model of health (Engel, 1977), one would consider not only physical health, but also emotional, social, and psychological well-being of older adults. Physical well-being is one facet of an individual's total well-being. Therefore, psychological well-being is just as important as physical well-being. The interrelatedness between one's social well-being, and one's physical well-being would also be considered according to this model. Therefore, health would be defined in accordance with the World Health Organization as a state of complete physical, mental, and social well-being, and not just the absence of disease. Complete health is an ideal, a goal that one continues to move toward, though never actually achieving.

Life-Span Developmental Perspective

Another expansion or shift is needed within health education. It is suggested that the paradigm of life-span developmental psychology and, therefore, developmental theories should be incorporated into the health education paradigm. "Led by a new paradigm, scientists adopt new instruments and new theories, and look in new places" (Kuhn, 1970, p. 111).

From a life-span developmental perspective, "development is now considered a continuous, dynamic and lifelong process of change" (Huyck & Hoyer, 1982, p. 4). Both the development of the individual and the family are considered to be lifelong processes. Development during adulthood may involve quantitative decline or positive change. The speed of decline may vary depending upon the particular process and life events (and environment) experienced. Changes in adulthood may also involve qualitative change as well as quantitative change. With this perspective, senescence is a subprocess of aging, and not synonomous with aging (Huyck & Hoyer, 1982; Papalla & Olds, 1986).

Chronological age is not an explanation for development, but a type of index. In fact, one could argue that an individual has many ages, such as biological, mental, and social age. The life-span developmentalist addresses the issue of nature-nurture interaction rather than age per se. A question of importance is how do particular experiences, the amount and timing of these experiences, interact with one's predisposition to develop particular behaviors and behavior change. From a life-span perspective, disease and aging are separate processes that interact; that is, as an individual ages, the probability of developing chronic diseases increase.

An example is given to illustrate the life-span developmental perspective to the health education domain. One important area of research in health education is determining effective stress reduction programs. How can the health educator help people cope with stressors? From the life-span perspective, one would ask questions such as the following: (a) Do older adults perceive and react to stressors in the same manner as younger adults? (b) How does the aging of the biological processes influence the individual's reactions to stressors? (c) Are there role or psychological process changes that influence reactions to stressors? (d) If so, do these changes have negative effects, or are there times when positive effects may occur? (e) Do older adults define active coping in the same way as younger adults?

Stressors are perceived differently depending upon one's stage of development. In the child developmental literature it had been assumed by the researchers that they knew what were distressors for children. However, research has shown that there can be disagreement between the adult's perspective, and the child's (Lewis, Siegel, & Lewis, 1984). Similarly, the younger adult researcher's perspective may not correspond to the older adult's perspective. For example, is transition to retirement a distressor for most people? Not necessarily. There are a number of ways of adjusting to retirement (Hornstein & Wapner, 1985). In conclusion, just as one would not provide the same health education for 4-year-olds as for 12-year-olds, so too, one would not necessarily have the same type or focus of intervention for 25-year-olds as for 75-year-olds.

The Perum and Bielby (1980) model of adult development is one of a number of models or theories within adult developmental psychology that has relevancy for the health educator. Perum and Bielby conceive of adult development as analogous to a set of disks in motion—similar to gears in a machine (Bee, 1987). As each gear moves at its own rate in a machine and has an effect upon the other gears in the machine, so too do changes in one part of one's life influence and cause change in another facet of one's life. During adulthood, physical changes occur (one type of "gear"); simultaneously, changes in family roles influence changes in work roles, and so on. Just as a machine works as one unit, though it may have many gears, so too an individual is perceived as one, even though there are many aspects to the one. In addition, the historical time in which adult development occurs is considered. The "synchrony" or "asynchrony" between the changing gears influence the smoothness of development.

With the wellness and life-span perspectives, the gerontological health educator would expand his or her focus from disease orientation to a focus on healthy aging. The positive aspects of wellness would be considered. Research would focus on what experiences (timing, type, and amount) are most effective at promoting health and well-being. The interaction between disease factors and aging factors would be evaluated. New research questions, such as the following, would be entertained: (a) What variables are present with older adults who are healthy and functioning? (b) How can health educators help older adults adapt to changes and/or successfully adapt to chronic diseases? (c) What interventions are best and most useful to educate older adults who are lower on the health-illness continuum (using Antonovsky's terminology)?

An example is given to illustrate the combination of wellness and life-span perspectives. As we age, changes occur in our sensory capabilities; for example, visual acuity declines. Eye glasses or contact lenses are needed, and usually utilized. Compensation results, and though a decline has occurred, one is able to function, that is, see (Atchley, 1987). Similarly, with these new perspectives, rather than only focusing on sensory decline in the absence of compensation, one would focus on how the older adult can utilize instruments or aids to compensate or maintain functioning. The focus is on adaptation to aging. Therefore, the gerontological health educator's role may be that of an educator of innovation; that is, the educator may provide programs that educate older adults about the availability, acceptance, and utilization of technological advancement. Some examples of these innovations are computer assistance in the home, telecommunication systems, cataract surgery, and new advances in hearing aids. This is in agreement with Green et al. (1980). They consider the health educator as one who "diffuses innovation."

New Approaches to Health Education

Therefore with these new perspectives, health education is defined as any combination of learning experiences that increases or changes behaviors (knowledge, beliefs, or attitudes) that: (a) promote wellness or optimal health, (b) decrease the risks of disease or impairment, (c) stop or slow down the effects of disease or a condition adverse to health, (d) return the individual to former health status or functioning given an adverse condition or disease, or (e) lead to successful adaption or functioning given an adverse condition or disease (that is, rehabilitation education) (e.g. Salamon, 1986). All aspects of well-being would be included. Gerontological health education is defined as health education that is designed to meet the health needs of older adults. The health education programs are designed from a life-span developmental perspective. Therefore, the goals of gerontological health education may be any of the above.

Measurements of success of health education programs would be expanded from morbidity and mortality rates to include quality of life measurements. Success would be measured by changes in indexes other than physical health, such as perceived health, happiness, mobility, or adaptation to devices. Health improvement would be measured not only by health status but by functional health and self-assessed health (see Engle and Granly, 1985–86). For example, success may be measured by an appropriate increase in the utilization of health services rather than a decrease in health services. This would be expected in programs that promote preventive screening procedures, such as yearly mammograms. In other programs, such as physical exercise programs, success may be measured by maintaining a certain level of strength rather than defining success as an increase in strength. As in the Kiyak preventive dentistry program, assessment of improvement may differ as related to the developmental and health status of the participants.

Comprehensive Gerontological Health Education

Also, there would be a shift to comprehensive gerontological health education. The comprehensive aspect is "borrowed" from the comprehensive school health education approach of Kolbe and Iverson (1985). Comprehensive school health programs consist of three components: health education, health services, and a healthy environment. "A comprehensive school health education program is comprehensive not only in content but in organization and implementation" (Florida Department of Education, 1980, cited in Kolbe and Iverson, 1984, p. 1103). There is coordination between services, health environments, and education. The educator may be any one of a number of significant people, including the teacher, school health aid, or pupil counselor.

Comprehensive gerontological health education would be provided within a number of different, already established institutions, such as, the Veterans Administration System, "Meals-on-Wheels" programs, senior centers, day centers, and extended care facilities. Education would be coordinated with other services. Unlike comprehensive school health education, however, the health educator is often an outsider to these systems. In the school setting, the health educator has a defined role as a teacher. In the health care systems for older adults, there often is not a defined occupational role as such. Consequently, the health educator may need to train health care providers, social workers, and administrators to become the direct health educators. In the Glanz, Marger, and Meehan study (1986), laypersons at senior centers were trained to become peer facilitators who then educated other center participants about stroke and stroke prevention. The key factor to this approach is that the gerontological health education is conducted in relation to other services, and not in isolation. A team approach is advocated. The consumer, the older adult, is an active participant in his or her own education.

Ecological Perspective

To provide effective comprehensive gerontological health education, an ecological perspective needs to be included within the health education paradigm. According to the ecological perspective, behavior is dependent upon the interaction of the person with the environment. The personal factors include one's attitudes, knowledge, skills, and behaviors; the environmental factors include the physical, social, and psychological environs. The environment has an effect upon the person, and the person reacts and affects the environment.

Accordingly, the gerontological health educator, when designing a health education program, would need to consider the interaction between the individual and the environment in which the program will occur. How the individual perceives and reacts to the environment, as well as how the environment reacts to the individual, would need to be assessed. The environment may be defined in a global manner, such as considering society, or more narrowly, by defining the environment at a particular site. Assessments would be made of both the physical and social environments. Therefore, the gerontological health educator may direct the health education to a variety of gatekeepers who are part of the "environment." The education, in fact, may not seem obviously related to the older adults' health behavior, but may be education about ageism, occupational role definitions of the gatekeepers, or assertive training for older adults. The gerontological health educator may function at training facilities and not at older adult centers or facilities at all.

More research is needed to determine how to best change society and the gatekeepers' attitudes about health and aging in order to implement comprehensive gerotological health education. Seefeldt (1987) found that preschoolers who regularly visited a nursing home, as compared to preschoolers who did not visit a nursing home, held more negative views toward the elderly, such as perceiving older people as more unfriendly and sick. Passive contact does not necessarily lead to positive attitude change. Evaluation of programs such as Leviton's Adult Health and Developmental Program (Leviton & Santa Maria, 1979) is needed to determine what effect active, positive interchange between generations has on the health and well-being of older and younger adults. Are programs that promote interrelatedness between generations better at changing attitudes? Should health care providers be trained not only at nursing home facilities, but also at senior citizen centers where they are able to have interchange with independent, healthy older adults? Answers to these questions are needed.

With the ecological orientation, before conducting a program in a particular setting, it may be necessary to analyze the organizational structure, and do a needs assessment of the staff. These analyses are more than an administrative diagnosis (Green et al., 1980). With an administrative diagnosis, the health educator determines what problems and resistance is expected in an organization. With the ecological orientation, in addition to determining the problems expected, the health educator assesses the bidirectional interactions and perceptions that occur. For example, Sigman (1985) points out that variation may occur between institutions such as some nursing homes oriented to the competent resident, whereas others are oriented to the resident who needs custodial care. Minkler (1984) discusses the lack of opportunity in certain institutions for residents to be effective responders. Some health care workers may define their occupational roles as the "provider," and receive rewards in "taking care of the patient." Though this is very altruistic, and needed in some cases, it may be counterproductive to the goals of a health education program. Other health care providers, especially direct care workers, may experience "rust-out." Pennington and Pierce (1985) suggest that staff may emotionally isolate themselves from residents because of boredom, which they label "rust-out." In some centers or resident facilities there also may be the paternalistic attitude: "I know what is best for you." The health educator's function, therefore, may be to educate the gatekeepers on how to expand their definitions of work to include the role of facilitator or health educator.

Ultimately, the recruitment and participation of older adults is needed for a successful gerontological health education program. Woodward and Wallston (1987) found that older adults desire less control concerning health-related decisions. The authors suggest that the lower locus of control is "mediated" by lower self-efficacy. According to Woodward and Wallston, the elderly perceive themselves as less effective and give up control to powerful others, such as physicians.

From an ecological perspective, the recruitment and participation of older adults is a complex issue. What aspects of the environment lead to participation? Schleser, West, and Boatwright (1986–87) found that the type of appeals utilized to recruit participants into a program can interact with the type of participants who initially come and continue in the program. The researchers compared strategies for recruiting community-dwelling elderly to a memory-training program. Three types of appeals—neutral, positive, and negative aspects of memory—were compared. Different approaches were used for each appeal. Schleser, West, and Boatwright found that older adults with different personality orientations were recruited with different appeals. For example, those who responded to the negative content message were more internally oriented.

One of the first studies that investigated active participation or control by older adults was conducted by Langer and Rodin (1976). This study was conducted in an institutional setting. In a more recent study, Franzke (1987) investigated the effects of assertive training for older adults living in the community. The participants in the study were volunteers who were either members of the American Association of Retired Persons, or attended nutrition centers in the community. Subjects were given a 6-week course on assertive training. Pre- and post-test measures were made on 2 self-reports, the Assertive Inventory, and the Burger Scale for Expressed Acceptance of Self. Franzke (1987) found the training to have an effect on self-reported changes for upper socio-economic older adults, but not for lower socio-economic older adults. The author suggests the need for more specialized assertive training for older adults. Considerations need to be made of the ethnicity (and, therefore, attitudes and norms) of the participants.

Slivinske and Fitch (1987) studied the effects of "control-enhancing interventions" for older adults living in retirement communities. A sample of 63 subjects from three retirement communities were randomly assigned to either an experimental condition, or control condition. The participants in the experimental group attended classes two times a week. The classes were on stress management, nutritional information, spirituality, and self-responsibility. They also attended physical education classes three times a week. (It is noted that the intervention could have been labeled a health education program.) The control group met together and played cards, talked about current events and other issues. There were no significant differences between the two groups for medical measures (such as muscular strength). The experimental group increased on measures of wellness and perceived control, whereas the control group decreased on these two sets of measurements. The attrition rate between pre- and post-tests was 32%. The authors hypothesize that at some retirement communities, there may be a decrease in the feelings of control and power among its residents. What aspects of retirement communities may lead to decreased participation? Would these results be found in all retirement communities? This study, as well as the other cited studies, highlight the need for more research about the ecological aspects of gerontological health education.

PART III

Theories

Within a particular paradigm a number of theories or models may coexist. A theory is defined as a "systematically related set of statements, including some lawlike generalizations, that is empirically testable" (Rudner, 1966, p. 10). Theories vary in their breadth and precision. The term model is sometimes used interchangeably with theory, sometimes as a synonym for metamodels, or sometimes as a general organizing framework to explain a process. There is a reciprocal relationship between theory and research. As hypotheses of theories are tested through scientific research, modifications are made to the theories. This in turn leads to new research.

An argument is made by some that theories are nonexistent in health education. Green (1984) suggests that health education "theory" is a hybrid of theories from other disciplines including anthropology, sociology, psychology, and epidemiology. The more popular models or theories, such as the Health Belief Model, have developed from social psychology theories. A very few studies have been conducted with older adults. The previously mentioned Woodward and Wallston study (1987) is one example. Another dominant area of health education research has been based upon conditioning models of learning. In a review of behavioral gerontological research, Ashley (1986–87) found that three-fourths of the studies were conducted in institutional settings. Ashley states that in the experimental behavioral research studies, the elderly are treated in a passive manner, and often not consulted about behavioral changes or types of reinforcements. Adult developmental psychology theories and models (which are within the life-span perspective) have not been dominant in the field of health education.

Having described these new perspectives for gerontological health education, I would like to describe a few developmental theories and models, and their relevancy to health education research. I have chosen cognitive theories and research, and family theories and research. Since the emphasis in health education is on "education," and the transmission of information, it is important to consider theories that describe adult information processing (perceptual, memory, learning intellectual, and cognitive processing) and techniques to modify these processes through education. Also, since health educators have had a great interest in the area of social support and health behavior change, the developmental aspects of social support within the family will be highlighted.

Cognitive Developmental Theories

Health education has not been tried with older adults because it has been assumed that cognitive or intellectual[2] functioning declines with age. Cummulative research suggest that this generalization is wrong. Factors, such as level of education, health status, and occupation during adulthood may influence cognitive functioning more than age per se. Whether intellectual change is positive or negative depends as much on what is measured and

---

[2]For brevity, I am using the terms cognitive and intellectual interchangeably. It is noted that researchers operationalize these terms differently.

how it is measured as when (age of person) it is measured (Huyck & Hoyer, 1982). In summarizing research on intellectual changes in adulthood (e.g., Schaie & Herzog, 1983) it is concluded that (a) intellectual declines generally don't occur until very old age, (b) declines vary between individuals, and within individuals varying with processes, (c) decline is more likely if speed is a factor, and (d) factors such as health correlate with decline rather than chronological age per se.

Denney (1985) hypothesizes that abilities that are optimally exercised (trained or performed) will decline later and less than abilities that are unexercised or untrained. Following from Denney's model and research, it can be concluded that adults may have abilities but not always use them; and secondly, that certain interventions may improve performance on problem-solving tasks for older adults.

Adult cognitive functioning may not only change quantitatively, but also qualitatively. Adult cognitive theorists, such as Labouvie-Vief (1980), argue that the nature of adult thinking is different from that of children and adolescents. Research indicates that adults may be more practical in their orientation to problem-solving than younger adults. Rather than thinking idealistically, the adult considers the impact that a decision will have on others. Both Schaie (1977) and Flavell (1979) theorize that adult thinking is strongly influenced by motivational factors, and by social awareness and attitudes. These motivational and social factors, such as the impact a decision may have on others, play an important role in one's decision-making process.

Jenkins's (1979) tetrahedral model of learning is a useful model to summarize the preceding discussion. Learning is dependent upon the characteristics of the learner (skills, knowledge, and attitudes), the nature of the materials (the modalities, the sequencing of material), the learning activity, and the criterion task (recall, transfer, recognition). With Jenkins' model, it is assumed that the ecology of the learning environment influences the learning that will occur.

Therefore, the gerontological health educator would want to consider each facet of the model when developing a relevant program for the elderly to ensure a "good match between the individual and the educational intervention." The educator may want to change the individual in relation to the environment, change the environment in relation to the individual, change both, or select a new environment for the learning to occur (Berg & Sternberg, 1985).

An application of these models is made to patient education. In order for patients to comply with recommendations they first must attend to the information given, and commit the information to memory. Later, they must be able to retrieve or recall the information at the correct time. Even though they may recall the information, they may not comply because of barriers, motivational or social factors.

It is hypothesized that patient education for older adults is likely to take place in an ecologically adverse learning environment. The patient is likely to be told in a short period of time emotionally disturbing information, such as "you have diabetes," that may require major life-style changes. A large amount of information, especially information about medications, may be given in a short period of time. Unfamiliar or technical terminology may be used. In addition, as stated earlier, the health care provider may hold stereotypes about aging, and interact negatively with the older patients. Rost and Roter (1987) found that 59% of older adults recalled medical information when interviewed immediately following their medical visits. They reported that 2.8 medications were newly prescribed or changed. Of the sample, 52% failed to recall life-style changes. It is noted that the average years of formal education for the sample was less than 8 years. Rost and Roter found a correlation between recall and patient-physician communication, and a negative correlation between number of medications and recall. Rost and Roter (1987) suggest that the communication style of the physician influences recall.

In addition, knowledge, attitude, and motivational factors of the "patient" may not be indexed. What is the patient's understanding of the illness? What impact will the recommendations have on the patient's spouse or children? How will the behavior change impact on the total well-being of the individual? For example, a patient may not perform breast self-examination for a variety of reasons. She may not know how, she may believe that it is not an effective technique, or she may not feel comfortable in touching her body. She may be willing to take a risk since she sees herself near the end of her life, and/or she may not want to discover a problem for fear of ending up being a burden to her family. A number of motivational and social factors may be operating at the same time.

Also, the modality of presentation, another important factor, may not be considered. Typically, information is presented orally, and only once. Clearly, this is not the best method. The information may never even be attended to, much less recalled. If reading material is given to the patient, the readability level may not be matched to the reading level of the patient. Also, illustrations and examples may not be relevant to the interests and life-style of the older patient. Certainly, when developing effective patient education programs and materials, complex multiple factors need to be considered.

An important avenue of research is delineating what are effective follow-up patient education techniques. How effective are follow-up interventions, such as telephone calls, taped messages, charts, videotapes, and so forth, on increasing recall and compliance? How effective is coordinating information given by the physician with information given by the pharmacist? There is a need to select new environments for patient education, environments that are more condusive to learning. It need not be assumed that all patient education takes place during the medical visit. As just described, this may be the worst environment for it to occur. Also, it is important to consider the perspective of the patient when designing the follow-up interventions.

Family Research and Theories

Just as the individual changes in adulthood, so too does the family. Much of family research and theory has focused on young children and their parents, such as the attachment between infant and mother. Only recently have the multiple "dialectical" relationships between family members been investigated. Due to a number of factors, such as increased life expectancy, adult developmental theorists have begun to research the multidimensional, interactive relationships between parent-adult child, grandparent-grandchild, adult siblings, and spousal relationships.

Duvall (1977) describes stages in the family life cycle. The last stage is called the Aging Family Stage in which one or both spouses is/are retired. The developmental tasks of adjusting to aging, coping with widowhood, and retirement are tasks that are prominent during this stage. Troll, Miller, and Atchley (1979) describe the "adult family" as a modified extended family. Though adult children usually do not live with their parents, the parent-child relationship of closeness is maintained. Adult children often visit their older parents (and vice versa), or they communicate regularly. Parents of adult children may continue to give financial support to the families of their adult child, even into middle age of the adult child. Conversely, adult children often help their parents in time of need. Certainly, there is a type of relationship or attachment between parent and adult child (Kahn & Antonucci, 1980). However, it is a much different relationship than between parent and young child.

Grandparenting styles are diverse and vary with the sex of the grandparent, sex of the grandchild, age of the grandparent, and age of the grandchild. Neugarten and Weinstein (1964) describe five styles of grandparenting: (a) the formal style, (b) the fun-seeking style, (c) the surrogate-parent style, (d) the reservoir of family wisdom style, and (e) the distant figure style. Within some ethnic groups in the United States, grandparents may play a significant role in the life of their grandchildren, and provide strong support for their children. Troll (1980; 1983) suggests that grandparents are "family watch-dogs" who provide support during family crises.

The intergenerational relationships and support between family members are dependent upon the type of life events, the timing of these life events, and the ethnic-cultural roles assigned to family members. The timing of the birth of children will influence the future relationships between generations, as each of the nuclear families age. For example, individuals who were 20 years old when they had their children will be entering the "old-old" age group of over 85, when their children will be entering the "young-old" age group of 65. Both the young-old and old-old adults may turn to their middle-aged grandchildren for assistance. Indeed, the middle-aged female child, whether daughter or daughter-in-law, is often the person who provides support to aging parents (Hagestad, 1984). Changes in family size, occupational roles for women, marriage-divorce rates, and social roles within ethnic groups highlight the fact that the relationships in the modified extended family are changing and varied.

For gerontological health educators, an important issue to consider is the social support provided by the family. In general, social support for changing health behavior is correlated with a positive change in behavior, though this is a complex relationship. Krause (1987) found that satisfaction of support correlated with self-rated health, but frequency of support did not. Also, if social obligation or problems are tied with the social support, the social support may not be correlated with positive health.

Social support may be emotional, informational, financial, providing care, or helping perform a behavior (Levitt, Antonucci, Clark, Ratton, & Finley, 1986). Important research questions are: (a) Who provides support for health education? (b) What types of support are given? (c) How can the social support of the gatekeepers in the family be elicited by the health educator?

To illustrate the above, health education concerning divorce will be discussed in relationship to social support provided by grandparents. Since grandparents are the watchdogs of the family, what effect does the divorce of a child have on older parents? How does it affect grandparenting relationships? In a very interesting descriptive study, Johnson and Barer (1987) found that multiple marriages of adult children may actually expand the number of kinship relationships. Mothers of sons may maintain their relationships with their daughters-in-law since the daughters-in-law often had custody of their grandchildren. Expansion of kinship relationships to step-siblings and step-grandparents of their grandchildren occurred for the paternal grandmothers. Gerontological health educators may want to investigate the role of grandparents as sources of support for their children and grandchildren. In addition, the health educator may want to investigate the needs and types of health education needed by the grandparents in helping them cope with the changes in the modified extended family. This example illustrates how gerontological health education may be broad in scope and intergenerational. Also, this illustration highlights the importance that the health needs of the older adult are not considered in isolation but as they relate to the needs of the rest of the family.

Research Methods and Statistics Issues

Just as a change in paradign will influence the theories a researcher utilizes, so too does it influence research sampling, methods, and designs. In this section, highlights of a few important research issues for gerontological health education are given.

When conducting research among older adults, the first factor to consider is the heterogeneity of the sample. When disseminating information about a study, it is necessary to give more specific and detailed descriptions of the older sample. From a developmental perspective, it is insufficient to simply say that the sample was aged. When was the sample taken? What was the health status of the sample? There is a very important need to sample community-dwelling and healthy older adults for health education research as well as institutional-dwelling older adults. In particular, some populations such as rural dwelling older adults have been underrepresented in studies. If samples are made at institutional settings, detailed descriptions of the institutions need to be provided. The importance of this was described in the ecological perspective section of this chapter.

There is no easy solution to controlling for the health status of an older adult sample (Siegler, Nowlin, & Blumenthal, 1980). It is known to be one of the most important factors that correlates with learning. One procedure is to vary or block on health status of the population. For example, the effectiveness of a pharmacological education program could be determined across a sample of older adults with diabetes compared to a sample with hypertension; both could be compared to a control sample. The interaction of the subject factor of disease category with the intervention could be assessed.

From a developmental perspective, another major factor to consider when doing research is cohort effects. A cohort is a group of individuals who share common historical, cultural, societal, physical, and/or biological events. The age range within a cohort may vary between studies. When doing cross sectional research, that is, comparing older and younger subjects, cohort and age factors are often confounded. Differences between age groups may be due to age differences or other factors, such as level of education.

It can be argued that the elderly consist of two cohorts, the young-old, about 65 to 80 years old, and the old-old, those over 80 years of age. (These two cohorts differ on a number of factors including, ratio of females to males, chronic diseases, historical events experienced, and so forth). Therefore, depending upon the research and hypotheses, the researcher may want to consider the elderly as two cohorts. For example, because there are differences in social networks between the two groups, the researcher may want to limit the age span of the sample to ensure more within-cell homogeneity.

The cohort factor is most important when planning gerontological health education for the future. The middle-aged adult of today, cohort born in 1940, has had many different historical events including differences in access to health education as compared to the present older adult cohort born in 1917. (It is noted that there are a number of possible middle-aged cohorts.) The gerontological health education of the future may be quite different (certainly, I hope, more) than that now provided. There is a need for longitudinal and/or time sequential studies to anticipate the needs of young and middle-aged adults.

The design of a study is dictated by the questions posed; that is, whether the researcher wants to (a) describe health behaviors (knowledge or attitudes); (b) predict these behaviors; (c) or control or change these behaviors. Most research has been descriptive. There is a need for more experimental or quasi-experimental studies with control groups. The fundamental question of determining effectiveness of programs cannot be determined adequately without at least some studies that involve control groups. The Hunt and Roll study (1987) is an excellent example of a study that employed a control group with a random assignment of subjects to conditions. The researchers were interested in determining effective interventions that could lessen the effects of relocation. Before intervening with older adults who were experiencing the problems of relocation, they sampled from volunteers who were healthy and ambulatory, and not actually being relocated. By conducting their study in this manner, they had more control over the setting and manipulations.

There is also the need for multiple testing over time (quasi-experimental with some variation of time). This is especially important with research with older adults because factors such as health status or social support may change during the time period. Multiple posttesting can help to determine if refresher intervention is needed or helpful.

The particular statistical analyses that are used to analyze the data are determined by the design of the research study and the sampling procedures. In this chapter, I have suggested the need for multiple measures over time.

Many of the variables are correlated. Therefore, multiple regression analyses, such as path analysis, are needed. Also, I would suggest more nonparametric analyses of qualitative data.

Developmentally, instruments (including questionnaires) may be reacted to differently depending upon one's age or cohort. The person interviewing, the particular questionnaire used, the questions posed, or the mode of presentation may cause the instruments to vary in reliability and/or validity. The previous discussion about stressors illustrates this problem.

Comparability of instruments over age is one of the most difficult methodological issues to control for when conducting developmental research. One partial solution is to utilize two instruments in a study, a standardized instrument that has been used with many samples, and a more specific program-related and population-derived instrument. Procedures analogous to that used in cross-cultural research are recommended. Berry (1969) describes the emic-etic methodologies in cross-cultural research. According to Berry, the emic instrument or questionnaire is derived from the population's own conceptualization, and not imposed by the "outside" researcher. The etic approach is imposed from the outsider's perspective. Therefore, using the emic approach in a health education study, particular items or concepts are elicited from an independent sample of older adults in the population. For example, it may be found that adults may define active coping as praying (an emic definition), but the researcher may define praying as passive coping (see Conway, 1985, for descriptions of types of coping and population definitions of stress). The relevancy of defining health from both the emic and etic approach is obvious. For example, Blazer, Hughes, and George (1987) suggest that the traditional DSM III categories do not define adequately "depressive elderly in the community." There is the need for population derived definitions of depression.

Another methodological problem to consider is the lack of familiarity with an instrument or mode of presentation. This problem is especially important for older subjects who did not grow-up with taking tests, or interacting with computers. These factors that are part of the experiment may mask the effectiveness of the experimental manipulation. However, it is important that the researcher not summarily discard a mode of presentation or procedure because the population may need some training. Data, especially daily behaviors such as taking medications, may be more accurately and more easily gathered with the use of a new procedure. For example, it may be easier and more accurate for an individual with arthritis to input data into a computer than to write it down in a diary. Therefore, the researcher may need to allow time for familiarity training with procedures prior to the actual study.

The final methodological issue is the most important because it is also an ethical issue. This issue centers on the welfare of the participants both during a study and after. Since many studies are conducted in passive inducing environments (using Minkler's terminology) the factor of voluntary participation in a study is questionable. Initially, the study may have to be done with a voluntary, community-dwelling sample that is less vulunerable. An example of such a study is the previously mentioned Hunt and Roll (1987) study. I strongly believe that the researcher needs to anticipate and consider what will happen to the participants, especially the control group, after the study is completed. It is important that the researcher plan how an effective program will be continued after he or she has left. This issue is most important when the study is conducted in an institutional setting. In some cases the researcher may do this by helping the group or agency acquire funding from government or private sources. Or the researcher may "transfer power" to participants or staff by directly training the members or staff. Videotapes or manuals may be made available. In some cases, the researcher may have to decide not to conduct the study at that time or place.

CONCLUSION

I began this paper by stating that the need for health education for older adults is expanding. Older adults are living longer than ever before with life expectancies of 15 or more years. It is not only important but necessary that society provide for an improved quality of life for its older members.

I have suggested that a change in perspective occur. Gerontological health education has been proposed as an alternative to the existing framework. The positive aspects of wellness and aging have been combined. This chapter has highlighted the complexity of gerontological health education. It is multileveled and multifaceted. Many more research questions have been raised than answered in this chapter. Certainly, this area of health education is in its infancy.

For an adoption of this change to gerontological health education, it is paramount that health educators be trained and perform a greater role in the gerontology field (which includes geriatrics). However, just as the paradigm of health education needs to be expanded, so too does the gerontology paradigm need to be expanded to include the health education orientation. Certainly, health promotion changes, such as changes in laws, need to occur for the expansion of health education into the gerontology field. Fortunately, these changes have begun to occur. Demonstration projects and centers on wellness and health promotion for the elderly have begun to be funded by the federal government. Associations and organizations, such as the American Association of Retired Persons, are initiating consumer awareness and advocacy programs for the elderly.

Therefore, quality research is needed to determine what are effective health education programs for the elderly. The time is right for health educators to play a dominant role in designing and evaluating health education for the elderly. The time is right for the merging of health education with gerontology since the possibility of improved health and well-being is an achievable goal for all of us whether we are 9 years old or 90 years old.

REFERENCES

American Association of Retired Persons (1987). *Ageline: A Database on Middle Age and Aging*. Washington, DC: American Association of Retired Persons.

Antonovsky, A. (1979). *Health, Stress, and Coping*. San Francisco: Jossey-Bass.

Antonovsky, A. (1984). The sense of coherence as a determinant of health. In J. Matarazzo, S. Weiss, J. Herd, N. Miller, & S. Weiss (Eds.), *Behavioral Health: A Handbook of Health Enhancement and Disease Prevention* (pp. 114–129). New York: John Wiley & Sons.

Ashley, P. (1986–87). Procedural and methodological parameters in behavioral-gerontological research: A review. *International Journal of Aging and Human Development, 24*(3), 189–229.

Atchley, R. (1987). *Aging: Continuity and Change* (pp. 19–23). Belmont, CA: Wadsworth Publishing Co.

Bastida, E. (1987). Sex-typed age norms among older Hispanics. *The Gerontologist, 27,* 59–65.

Baum, H. M. (1987). National trends in stroke-related mortality. *The Gerontologist, 27*(3), 293–300.

Bee, H. (1987). *The Journey of Adulthood*. New York: MacMillan Publishing Co.

Berg, C., & Sternberg, R. (1985). A triarchic theory of intellectual development during adulthood. *Developmental Review, 5*(4), 334–370.

Berry, J. (1969). On cross-cultural comparability. *International Journal of Psychology, 4*(2), 119–128.

Blazer, D., Hughes, D., & George, L. (1987). The epidemiology of depression in an elderly community population. *The Gerontologist, 27*(3), 281–287.

Braithwaite, V., Gibson, D., & Holman, J. (1985–86). Age stereotyping: Are we oversymplifying the phenomenon? *International Journal of and Human Development, 22*(4), 315–325.

Conway, K. (1985). Coping with the stress of medical problems among black and white elderly. *International Journal of Aging and Human Development, 21*(1), 39–48.

Denney, N. (1985). A review of life-span research with the twenty question task: A study of problem-solving ability. *International Journal of Aging and Human Development, 21*(3), 161–173.

De Tullio, P., Eraker, S., Jepson, C., Becker, M., Fujimoto, E., Diaz, C., Loveland, R., and Strecher, V. (1986). Patient medication instruction and provider interactions: Effects on knowledge and attitudes. *Health Education Quarterly, 13*(1), 51–60.

Duvall, E. (1977). *Marriage and Family Development* (5th ed.). New York: Lippincott.

Engel, G. (1977). The need for a new medical model: A challenge for biomedicine. *Science, 196,* 129–136.

Engle, V., & Granly, M. (1985–86). Self-assessed and functional health of older women. *International Journal of Aging and Human Development, 22*(4), 301–313.

Everly, G. (1985). Time management training: Overcoming a major barrier to occupational health promotion. In G. Everly & R. Feldman (Eds.), *Occupational Health Promotion* (pp. 221–230). New York: John Wiley & Sons.

Flavell, J. (1979). Metacognition and cognitive monitoring: A new area of psychological inquiry. *American Psychologist, 34,* 906–911.

Florida Department of Education. (1980). Cited in L. Kolbe & D. Iverson (1985), Comprehensive school health education programs. In J. Matarazzo, S. Weiss, J. Herd, N. Miller, & S. Weiss (Eds.), *Behavioral Health: A Handbook of Health Enhancement and Disease Prevention* (pp. 1094–1116). New York: John Wiley & Sons.

Franzke, A. (1987). The effects of assertive training on older adults. *The Gerontologist 27*(1), 13–16.

Glanz, K., Marger, S., & Meehan, E. (1986). Evaluation of a peer education stroke education program for the elderly. *Health Education Research, 1*(2), 121–130.

Green, L. (1984). Health education models. In J. Matarazzo, S. Weiss, J. Herd, N. Miller, & S. Weiss. (Eds.), *Behavioral Health: A Handbook of Health Enhancement and Disease Prevention* (pp. 181–194). New York: John Wiley & Sons.

Green, L., Kreuter, M., Deeds, S., & Partridge, K. (1980). *Health Education: A Diagnostic Approach.* Palo Alto., CA: Mayfield Publishing Co.

Greene, M., Hoffman, S., Charon, R., & Adelman, R. (1987). Psychosocial concerns in the medical encounter: A comparison of the interactions of doctors with their old and young patients. *The Gerontologist, 27,* 164–168.

Hagestad, G. (1984). The continuous bond: A dynamic, multigenerational perspective on parent-child relations between adults. In M. Perlmutter (Ed.), *Minnesota Symposia on Child Psychology* (Vol. 17, pp. 106–119), Hillsdale, NJ: Lawrence Erlbaum & Associates.

Hoffand, B., Smyer, M., Wetle, T., & Walter, A. (1987). Linking research and practice: The fellowship program in applied gerontology. *The Gerontologist, 27*(1), 39–45.

Hornstein, G., & Wapner, S. (1985). Modes of experiencing and adapting to retirement. *International Journal of Aging and Human Development, 21*(4), 291–315.

Hunt, M., & Roll, M. (1987). Simulation in familiarizing older people with an unknown building. *The Gerontologist, 27*(2), 169–175.

Huyck, M., & Hoyer, W. (1982). *Adult Development and Aging.* Belmont, CA: Wadsworth Publishing Co.

Jenkins, J. J. (1979). Four points to remember: A tetrahedral model of memory experiments. In L. S. Cermak & F. Craik (Eds.), *Levels of Processing in Memory.* Hillsdale, NJ: Lawrence Erlbaum & Associates.

Johnson, C., & Barer, B. (1987). Marital instability and the changing kinship network of grandparents. *The Gerontologist, 27*(3), 330–335.

Kahn, R., & Antonucci, T. (1980). Convoys over the life course: Attachment, roles, and social support. In P. B. Baltes & O. Brim, (Eds.), *Life-Span Development and Behavior* (Vol. 3, pp.). New York: Academic Press.

Kane-Williams, E. (1987). Cross-cultural program implementation: Health promotion for Black, Hispanic, and Asian older persons. Presented at the Society for Public Health Education, New Orleans.

Keyes, K., Bisno, B., Richardson, J., & Mueston, A. (1987). Age differences in coping, behavioral dysfunctioning, and depression following colostomy surgery. *The Gerontologist, 27,* 182–184.

Kime, R., Schlaadt, R., & Tritsch, L. (1977). *Health Instruction: An Action Approach.* Englewood Cliffs, NJ: Prentice-Hall, Inc.

Kiyak, H. (1984). Oral health promotion for the elderly. In J. Matarazzo, S. Weiss, J. Herd, N. Miller, & S. Weiss, *Behavioral Health: A Handbook of Health Enhancement and Disease Prevention* (pp. 967–975). New York: John Wiley & Sons.

Koh, J., & Bell, W. (1987). Korean elders in the United States: intergenerational relations and living arrangements. *The Gerontologist, 27,* 66–71.

Kolbe, L., & Iverson, D. (1985). Comprehensive school health education programs. In J. Matarazzo, J. S. Weiss, J. Herd, N. Miller, & S. Weiss (Eds.), *Behavioral Health: A Handbook of Health Enhancement and Disease Prevention* (pp. 114–129). New York: John Wiley & sons.

Krause, N. (1987). Satisfaction with social support and self-rated health in older adults. *The Gerontologist, 27*(3), 301–308.

Krauss, I. (1980). Between and within-group comparisons in aging research. In L. Poon (Ed.), *Aging in the 1980s: Psychological Issues* (pp. 542–551). Washington, DC: American Psychological Association, Inc.

Kuhn, T. (1970). *The Structure of Scientific Revolutions.* Chicago, IL: The University of Chicago Press.

Kushman, J., & Freeman, B. (1986). Service consciousness and service knowledge among older Americans. *International Journal of Aging and Human Development, 23*(3), 217–237.

Labouvie-Vief, G. (1980). Beyond formal operations: Uses and limits of pure logic in life-span development, *Human Development, 23,* 141–161.

Langer, E., & Rodin, J. (1976). The effects of choice and enhanced personal responsibility in an institutional setting. *Journal of Personality and Social Psychology 34*(2), 191–198.

Lasoski, M., & Thelen, M. (1987). Attitudes of older and middle-aged persons toward mental health intervention. *The Gerontologist, 27,* 289–292.

Leviton, D., & Santa Maria, L. (1979). The adult's health and developmental program: Descriptive and evaluative data. *The Gerontologist, 19*(6), 534–543.

Levitt, M., Antonucci, T., Clark, M., Ratton, J., & Finley, G. (1985–86). Social support and well-being: Preliminary indicators based on two samples of the elderly, *International Journal of Aging and Human Development 21*(1), 61–77.

Lewis, C., Siegel, J., & Lewis, M. (1984). Feeling bad: Exploring sources of distress among pre-adolescent children. *American Journal of Public Health, 74*(20), 117–122.

Lilienfeld, A., & Lilienfeld, D. (1980), *Foundations of Epidemiology* (2nd ed.). New York: Oxford University Press.

Luboudrov, S. (1987). Congressional perceptions of the elderly: The use of stereotypes in the legislative process. *The Gerontologist, 27,* 77–81.

Matarazzo, J. (1984). Behavioral health: A 1990 challenge for health services professions. In J. Matarazzo, S. Weiss, J. Herd, N. Miller, & S. Weiss, (Eds.), *Behavioral Health: A Handbook of Health Enhancement and Disease Prevention* (pp. 3–30). New York: John Wiley & Sons.

Minkler, M. (1984). Health promotion in long-term care: Contradiction in terms? *Health Education Quarterly, 11,* 77–89.

Mitterness, L. (1987). The management of urinary incontinence. *The Gerontologist, 27,* 185–193.

Nelson, E., McHugo, G., Schnurr, P., Devito, C., Roberts, E., Simmer, J., & Zubkoff, W. (1984). Medical self-care education for elders: A controlled trial to evaluate impact. *American Journal of Public Health, 74*(12), 1357–1362.

Neugarten, B., & Weinstein, K. (1964). The changing American grandparent. *Journal of Marriage and the Family, 26,* 199–204.

Papalia, D., & Olds, S. (1986). *Human Development.* New York: McGraw—Hill.

Pennington, R., & Pierce, W. (1985). Observation of empathy of nursing-home staff: a predictive study. *International Journal of Aging and Human Development, 21*(4), 281–290.

Perum, P., & Bielby, D. (1980). Structure and dynamics of the individual life course. In K. W. Back (Ed.), *Life Course: Integrative Theories and Exemplary Populations* Boulder, CO: Westview Press.

Prohaska, T., Keller, M., Leventhal, E., & Leventhal H. (1987). Impact of symptoms and aging attribution on emotions and coping. *Health Psychology, 6*(6), 495–514.

Quinn, P., & Keznikoff, M. (1985). The relationship between death anxiety and the subjective experience of time in the elderly. *International Journal of Aging and Human Development, 21*(3), 197–210.

Rakowski, W., Hickey, T., & Dengiz, A. (1987). Congruence of health and treatment perceptions among older patients and providers of primary care. *International Journal of Aging and Human Development, 25,* 63–77.

Ray, D., McKinney, K., & Ford, C. (1987). Differences in psychologists ratings of older and younger clients. *The Gerontologist, 27,* 82–91.

Rosenwaike, I., & Dolinsky, A. (1987). The changing determinants of the growth of the extremely aged. *The Gerontologist, 27,* 275–280.

Rost, K., & Roter, D. (1987). Predictors of recall of medical regimens and recommendations for lifestyle change in elderly patients. *The Gerontologist, 27,* 510–515.

Rudner, R. (1966). *Philosophy of Social Science.* Englewood Cliffs, NJ: Prentice-Hall, Inc.

Salamon, M. (1986). The matrix of care: A heuristic for assessment and placement. *The International Journal of Aging and Human Development, 23*(3), 207–216.

Schaie, K. (1977). Toward a stage theory of adult cognitive development. *International Journal of Aging and Human Development, 8,* 129–138.

Schaie, K., & Herzog, C. (1983). Fourteen-year cohort sequential analyses of adult intellectual development. *Developmental Psychology, 19*(4), 531–543.

Schleser, R., West, R., & Boatwright, L. (1986–87). A comparison of recruiting strategies for increasing older adults initial entry and compliance in a memory training program. *International Journal of Aging and Human Development, 24*(1), 55–66.

Seefeldt, C. (1987). The effects of preschoolers visits to a nursing home. *The Gerontologist, 27*(2), 228–232.

Shakespeare, W. *As You Like It.* In Wright (Ed.) (1939), *The Complete Works of William Shakespeare.* Garden City, New York: Garden City Books.

Siegler, I. Nowlin, J., & Blumenthal, J. (1980). In L. Poon (Ed.), *Aging in the 1980s: Psychological Issues* (pp. 599–612). Washington, DC: American Psychological Association.

Sigman, S. (1985). Conversational behavior in two health care institutions for the elderly. *International Journal of Aging and Human Development, 21*(2), 137–154.

Slivinske, L. R., & Fitch, V. (1987). The effects of control enhancing: Interventions on the well-being of elderly individuals living in retirement communities. *The Gerontologist, 27*(2), 176–181.

Troll, L. (1980). Grandparenting. In L. Poon, (Ed.), *Aging in the 1980s: Psychological Issues* (pp. 475–481). Washington, DC: American Psychological Association.

Troll, L. (1983). Grandparents: the family watchdogs. In T. H. Brubaker (Ed.), *Family Relationships in Later Life* (pp. 63–74). Beverly Hills: Sage.

Troll, L. Miller, S., & Atchley, R. (1979). *Families in Later Life.* Belmont, CA: Wadsworth.

U.S. Bureau of the Census. (1984). *Current Population Reports P-23, No. 138, Demographic and Socioeconomic Aspects of Aging in the United States.* Washington, DC: U.S. Government Printing Office.

Webster's New Collegiate Dictionary (1974). Springfield, MA: G. & C. Merrian Co.

Wilson-Pessano, S., Scamagas, P., Arsham, G. Chardon, L., Coss, S., German, D., & Hughes, G. (1987). An evaluation of approaches to asthma self-management education for adults: The AIR/Kaiser-Permamente Study. *Health Education Quarterly, 14*(3), 333–343.

Wison, C., & Netting, F. (1987). Comparison of self and health professionals' ratings of the health of community-based elderly. *International Journal of Aging and Human Development, 25*(1), 11–25.

Wolfe, S. (Ed.). (1988). Poor health care for poor Americans. *Health Letter, 4*(1), 1–6.

Woodward, N., & Wallston, B. (1987). Age and health care beliefs: Self-efficacy as a mediator of low desire for control. *Psychology and Aging, 2*(1), 3–8.

Zopf, P. (1986). *America's Older Population.* Houston, TX: Cap and Gown Press, Inc.

13

PATIENT EDUCATION IN PRIMARY CARE SETTINGS: A REVIEW OF THE LITERATURE

Janet Fraser Hale
Jerrold S. Greenberg

Health care costs are rising dramatically. The leading causes of death have changed from infectious and communicable diseases to life-style related diseases. There is a national effort to promote disease prevention and health promotion and the suggestion that patient education be incorporated into the primary care medical setting. Yet, the implications and problems associated with this suggestion have not been adequately explored. This manuscript identifies the numerous and diverse difficulties encountered in patient education in primary care settings, including: lack of appropriate financing; lack of strong scientific evidence of the benefits of health promotion/disease prevention programs; difficulties in making behavior changes; education and territorial concerns of health care providers; and the attitudes among health care providers, health care consumers, and third party payers. Additionally, current efforts and proposed methods for promoting health and preventing disease in the medical/health care arena are discussed.

This chapter presents a review of the literature relating to the history and development of health promotion and disease prevention efforts in the primary care setting, the concerns and obstacles which hinder health promotion and disease prevention efforts in these settings, and examples of both current and proposed methods for promoting health and preventing disease in the medical/health care arena.

HIGH COST OF HEALTH CARE

Health care costs are rising dramatically (Green, 1985). In 1960, medical care expenditures in the United States were $26.9 billion (5.3% of the Gross National Product, GNP). In 1980, these expenses had increased to $234.4 billion (9.4% of the GNP). In 1985, 10% of the GNP was spent on illness care costs (Green, 1985; Kaplan, 1985). Health care costs related to the top four killers continue to increase significantly. The median cost of treating one case of lung cancer in Wisconsin was estimated at $50,000. Smoking related cancer treatment costs in Wisconsin total over $70 million per year (Rentmeester, 1984). Such medical care expenditures have resulted in significant interest in not only determining strategies to curb this growth but developing strategies to improve individual health and well-being through health promotion and disease prevention efforts as well.

MORBIDITY AND MORTALITY STATISTICS

Technology for curing and caring has increased in complexity, with little impact on mortality rates. However, the leading causes of death have changed; infectious and communicable diseases have given way to life-style related causes of death (Green, 1985). As Dr. Brandt (1985) of The National Center for Health Promotion and Preventive Medicine stated:

> It is clear that the causes of many of our more common diseases are the direct result of our own behavior, such as a sedentary life-style, poor diet and weight control, abuse of alcohol and drugs, and smoking. . . . Yet we still seem to be more concerned with treating diseases than preventing their occurrence. Although it is widely known that many diseases can be directly linked to the way we work and live, the emphasis has only slowly begun to shift from reacting to illness to promoting health. (p. 1)

Seventy-five percent of the deaths in the United States result from the degenerative conditions of heart disease, stroke, and cancer with accidents ranking as the most frequent cause of death from age one through the early forties. Environmental hazards coupled with behavioral factors mete out a heavy toll on the people's health (U.S. Department of Health, Education, and Welfare, 1978; U.S. Department of Health, Education, and Welfare, 1980a). For the top three diseases contributing to premature mortality, life-style contributes 54% to heart disease, 37% to cancer, and 50% to cerebrovascular disease (Brandt, 1985); while life-style and the environment together contribute 64% to mortality (Yoder, Jones, & Jones, 1985). The need to reduce risk factors (whether they arise from the environment or personal behavior) is recognized as a necessary part of health care (Logsdon, Rosen, & Demak 1982).

NATIONAL EFFORTS 1965 TO PRESENT

The profound shift in causes of death from acute infections to chronic disease and accidents during this century, prompted the release of the United States' Surgeon General's reports on smoking and health and heralded a major national effort in disease prevention/health promotion. These reports, first released in 1964, initiated major national efforts to prevent nonsmokers from adopting smoking habits and to help smokers quit. In the early 1970s, the work of the President's Committee on Health Education resulted in the 1974 National Health Planning and Resources Development Act and the 1976 National Consumer Health Information and Health Promotion Act. These Acts focused on national and regional efforts in health education.

In 1973, in anticipation of the forthcoming emphasis on prevention at the federal level, the National Institutes of Health initiated a series of studies to review and evaluate the field of prevention. They identified the need for an age-specific preventive procedure for patient care as a replacement to the annual medical examination (Logsdon et al., 1982). The objectives of the national prevention strategy were to eliminate or reduce the incidence and prevalence of preventable factors that increase the risk of disease, and to promote and enhance the well-being of the public (USDHEW, 1978). In 1976, the Office of Disease Prevention and Health Promotion (ODPHP) of the Department of Health and Human Services was established and in 1979 ODPHP published *Healthy People, the Surgeon General's Report on Health Promotion and Disease Prevention* (USDHEW, 1979). *Healthy People* was the first federal document to describe a national commitment to improving the health of the United States population through disease prevention and health promotion activities. *Healthy People* identified national opportunities in prevention and established quantifiable goals for health improvements for people in five life stages by 1990 (Harrell, 1986; USDHEW, 1979). In 1980, these goals were translated into 200 achievable objectives and published as *Promoting Health Preventing Disease: Objectives for the Nation* (United States Department of Health and Human Services, 1981). It was recognized that achievement of these objectives required a coordinated effort of the government, the public, and the medical and health professions (USDHHS, 1980).

The next step was a conference specifically designed to acquaint representatives of 50 national organizations from health care settings, health professions, business, industry, voluntary organizations, and schools with the *Objectives for the Nation* and to encourage their participation in a coordinated effort to achieve those objectives by 1990. The results of this conference were published as *Prospects for a Healthier America: Achieving the Nation's Health Promotion Objectives* (USDHHS, 1984b). During the conference each of the groups acknowledged the importance of the objectives in their organization's goals, and suggested ways for the federal government and the private sector to cooperate to achieve the objectives.

With national focus, as well as supportive statistical data, emphasizing the need for life-style and behavior changes to reduce morbidity and mortality and to arrest the rising costs of health care—why is there still a problem?

THE PROBLEM

The difficulties encountered in health promotion/disease prevention efforts are numerous and diverse. These difficulties, or barriers, include: lack of appropriate financing; lack of strong scientific evidence of the benefits of health promotion/disease prevention programs; difficulties in making behavior changes; education and territorial concerns of health care providers; and the attitudes among health care providers, health care consumers, and third party payers. These barriers are explored in detail in the following discussion.

Financing Preventive Health Care

While verbal support at the federal and state levels has been expressed, adequate resources have not been provided to support health promotion program development, implementation, and evaluation.

Rentmeester (1984) stated:

> Government, by its nature, responds to crises and financially supports services that directly address problems and crises. Since wellness programs are focused primarily on keeping people healthy, and as such are future oriented, government is unable to fund programs which are not tangibly related to the present need for illness care. (p. 8)

There is an investment of greater funds in what is basically illness care health insurance than in programs for promoting health. There is a greater interest in the etiology of illness than in the dynamics of health (Yoder et al., 1985; Orlandi, 1987). Federal funding for health promotion/disease prevention programs has been minimal compared to that provided for the study and treatment of diseases—97 cents out of every health care dollar goes for treatment. Less than 2.5% of the national expenditure on health care has been for disease prevention and only 0.5% has been provided for health promotion activities (Polakoff, 1982).

This attitude is further evidenced by appropriations from the most current Congress at the time of this writing (the 99th Congress), which provided the Office of Disease Prevention and Health Promotion with $3.6 million, while the National Institutes of Health, with primarily an illness focus, received $6.18 billion (Barbour, 1987b).

Third Party Payment

With the decrease in federal funding for health promotion, third party payment by insurance companies is a likely potential funding source. However, this funding is unlikely to come about until preventive strategies are shown to have a major impact on health care costs and/or morbidity and mortality (USDHHS, 1984b; Orlandi, 1986). In theory, health promotion is consistent with the goals of long term cost containment, but current efforts are geared toward cost control in the short run. Reimbursement practices favor episodic, technical medical services in hospital settings (Fletcher, 1985; Nutting, 1986).

The issue of cost containment is central. Third party payers financed 68% of the total cost of personal health care in 1981. Employers account for 80% of private health insurance payments. Health care expenditures have grown at an average annual rate of 12.8% since 1965 (Logsdon & Rosen, 1984).

In an effort to contain costs, decreasing health insurance benefits and/or eliminating new benefits has been the action taken by employers and carriers. Many health insurance programs specifically *exclude* payment for preventive services, because preventive services do not fit the category of "unpredictable risk." Others limit first-dollar coverage with higher deductibles and coinsurance emphasizing technical care for illnesses after they have occurred (Roemer, 1984; Nutting, 1986). These types of actions appear to inhibit the possibilities of coverage for preventive care in the near future. Physicians (Logsdon & Rosen, 1984) and consumers (David & Boldt, 1980) believe physicians should incorporate preventive health care into their practices, but physicians indicate that the lack of third party reimbursement is a major obstacle (McGinnis, Moritsugu, & Roberts, 1982; McNamara, 1982; Relman, 1982; Weinberg & Andrus, 1982; Ford & Ford, 1983; Logsdon &

Rosen, 1984; Orleans, George, Houpt, & Brodie, 1985; Altekruse, 1986). Lack of third party reimbursement was listed as a major barrier to incorporating preventive health care into the practices of 64% of the primary care physicians who responded to a 1983 survey by Ford and Ford. Another survey reported that limited third party reimbursement was an obstacle to incorporating preventive health care into the practices of 25% of responding family practice physicians (Orleans et al., 1985). An even bleaker perspective was reported in a Massachusetts study, which found that less than one-third of the physicians believed reimbursement for time spent on health promotion would be very valuable (Wechsler, Levin, Idelson, Rohman, & Taylor, 1983).

The perspective of third party payers is that the reimbursement already provided should include health education activities, and they express additional concern that not enough research has been done to demonstrate the effectiveness and cost benefits of health education (Campbell & Valente, 1983).

Third parties will play an instrumental part in the future of health promotion should they decide to offer more liberal reimbursement for risk reduction practices. A crucial barrier would be removed and physicians would have a greater incentive to integrate increased health promotion efforts into their practices (Nutting, 1986). According to Altekruse (1986):

> The absence of third party compensation and other direct monetary support and incentives for preventive services are serious and idiosyncratic deficits in our present medical care system. However, compensation for preventive child health services is now required under insurance coverage in some states and evolving in others. These and other pending revisions in payment mechanisms can be counted on to create great, if not revolutionary, receptivity on the part of potential providers to recast themselves as preventive care practitioners. (p. 6)

Closely related to the lack of reimbursement for disease prevention/health promotion activities has been the lack of strong scientific evidence of the impact of these programs on morbidity and mortality.

Lack of Scientific Research to Support the Benefits of Disease Prevention/Health Promotion Activities

For many years there has been a dearth of sound scientific research available to support the specific outcomes of health promotion/disease prevention programs (Orlandi, 1987). Clinicians, therefore, have been less than interested in focusing on health promotion, especially given the lack of third party coverage (USDHEW 1980a). When the 1984 national conference of health related organizations met to plan how to reach the 1990 objectives, each of the groups identified the need for more formal evaluation of health promotion programs. Additionally, they advocated implementing a mechanism for more rapid dissemination of findings to health care providers and organizations (USDHHS 1984b).

According to *Living Well* (USDHEW 1980a), health promotion is defined as those methods utilized to augment physical and emotional well-being, to increase longevity and to enhance the quality of life. Disease prevention and health promotion can save individuals' lives and prolong their productive years, improve the quality of their lives, and save money through the prevention of disease. However, the lack of sound scientific research to support these outcomes is often cited by funding sources and clinicians as a reason for their lack of interest in funding and implementing health promotion activities (USDHEW, 1980a). While costs are quite apparent, benefits may not be evident except over the long term. The precise long term effects of health promotion are yet unknown and some well-meaning proponents have grossly exaggerated the benefits and set up false and unachievable expectations (Fletcher, 1985).

Cost-benefit analyses can be extremely useful in identifying indirect costs and to demonstrate that, in some cases, the total savings, direct and indirect, from such programs can be considerable (McGinnis, 1980). Additionally, it is reported that patients who participate in their own care have more reasonable expectations, share more responsibility for their care and are less likely to become involved in medical litigation (Brody, 1984; Prather, 1984). While substantial cost-savings from many prevention programs can be anticipated, these programs should be appreciated for their merits in reducing human suffering, and should be supported from that perspective as well as on economic grounds (McGinnis, 1980). Health educators should be aware of the possibility of a double standard—health education programs may be judged by rigorous scientific standards whereas medical interventions are approved on the basis of clinical experience and patient report (Bartlett, 1983). The Congressional Office of Technology Assessment reports that *at most* 30% of medical procedures are demonstrated to be effective. Even without a demonstrated increased effectiveness of programs, health educators should not allow requests for demonstration of effectiveness to be applied to patient education when they are not applied to other preventive and therapeutic treatments. Often requests for more data and more scientific evidence to support an intervention are merely a smoke screen or a polite way to say "no" (Bartlett, 1983). Associated with the lack of research-based support for many health promotion/disease prevention activities is the inherent difficulty related to changing life-styles and health habits that are not conducive to good health. Many of the activities required of human-kind to live in a more healthful manner demand significant adaptations and changes in habits/life-styles that have been firmly ingrained throughout an individual's life.

Difficulties in Changing Lifestyle/Health Behaviors

Lawrence Green (1980) defined health education as "any combination of learning experiences designed to facilitate voluntary adaptations of behavior conducive to health" (p. 2). The emphasis here is on the word *voluntary* and, as such, the difficulty of encouraging behavior change becomes apparent.

More than health risk education and behavioral change advice are needed to successfully modify behavioral risks (USDHEW 1979). Telling is not educating. Knowledge is necessary but not sufficient for changing behavior (La Vigne, 1980). Even in the case of therapeutic treatment of illness, the provision of information does not necessarily increase compliance (Becker, 1985) and most health behavior change programs have high failure rates (Weinberg & Andrus, 1982).

Although physicians do occupy a special status and authority, which helps them to persuade individuals to alter their habits (Jonas, 1981), patients need access to effective behavior change skills and assistance to replace unhealthy habits with healthy alternatives (Orleans et al., 1985). A variety of educational methods must be used to facilitate patient behavior. These include support, reinforcement, and involvement of peers, family, and/or significant others in the process (Campbell & Valente, 1983). Individual counseling and teaching are the most commonly used educational methods in clinical practice. This educational strategy is fine for information dissemination, but generally less effective for attitudinal and behavioral change. While highly individualized communication is possible, it is less efficient (and for certain problems, less effective) than group methods (La Vigne, 1980). It is the domain of the health educator to design a combination of methods that can be tailored to individual needs to promote a voluntary change in behavior. As Isbister (1976) stated, what is needed is "more health education done in a meaningful way by sensitive health educators" (p. 95).

The concept of health promotion moves the burden of responsibility for health from the health care provider to the consumer (Green, 1985). The challenge to individuals is to take personal responsibility for health through life-style modification. Brandt (1985) believes Americans are genuinely interested in improving their health as evidenced by their increased emphasis on exercise, nutrition, environmental health, and occupational safety. Factors impacting upon consumers' health behaviors include family, social, community, and cultural norms that are based on beliefs held by an individual regarding health and illness. Additionally, health behaviors are influenced by the amount and type of health information known to an individual, previous health habits and skills, and the amount of effort it takes to achieve a positive health outcome coupled with the specific information as to how to achieve results (Brandt, 1985). Unfortunately there is still a tendency among consumers to rely on health care providers for treatments and cures rather than behavioral advice (Orlandi, 1987).

The Medical Care Setting

With all of the national attention and focus on disease prevention and health promotion, the medical profession's silence has been conspicuous (Nutting, 1986). In addition to being fostered by the lack of third party reimbursement for their health education efforts, the general disinterest of physicians toward disease prevention and health promotion is inculcated during the medical education process, significantly contributing to their disinterest once in practice. This problem and others are explored in the ensuing discussion.

Medical Education Past and Present.   According to Jonas (1981), "there are two principle influences on how physicians work: how they are trained and how they are paid" (p. 700). Traditional medical education has not emphasized health promotion/disease prevention activities in the curriculum. The health promotion/disease prevention content areas have been specifically cited as lacking substance or even mention in many medical education programs. The difficulties encountered by physicians in providing health education to their patients are due to the lack of the inclusion of health education principles in the curriculum, the lack of knowledge of the complexity of and the skills necessary to change behavior, the lack of time to incorporate health education into medical care (the medical encounter is usually time-limited and structured for acute care), a lack of a value placed on the benefits of health promotion/disease prevention, and the cost of providing health education (Campbell & Valente, 1983; Nutting, 1986).

Medical education has been committed to diagnosis and treatment of disease (Jonas, 1981; Relman, 1982; Orlandi, 1987). Physicians have been educated to cure and may feel like personal and professional failures when cures are not possible (Green, 1985). Disease prevention concepts continue to have a weak foothold in the medical system (DeMuth, Fielding, Stunkard, & Hollander, 1986) and are seen by physicians as well as patients as peripheral to the main body of medicine (Relman, 1982).

Although preventive medicine has been a concern of medicine, it has received little emphasis (Barker & Jonas, 1981). Beginning in the 1970s, any health education that was included in medical school curricula was incorporated into preventive medicine (Barlett, 1984). However, even as recently as 1984, prevention received only 1.5% of the total teaching time in medical education curricula (Jonas, 1981) and as of 1985, prevention was still not a universally accepted area of medical curricula nationally or internationally (Scott & Neighbor, 1985).

Simpson and Wilson (1985) reported that the chairpersons of 124 accredited U.S. medical schools offered 484 different courses with prevention content. However, only 37% of these courses were required. Although 74% of the medical chairpersons said these types of courses should be required, 64% stated the curriculum was already too full to require these types of courses. Thirty-one percent of the medical school chairpersons listed lack of interest or support as a reason for not requiring courses on prevention (Simpson & Wilson, 1985).

As stated by McGinnis et al. in 1982:

> Diagnosis and treatment will, in any foreseeable future, continue to be the primary responsibility of the physician. Thus, medical students must continue to be taught, and to learn, an ever-increasing body of knowledge and repertoire of diagnostic and treatment skills. (p. 242)

Current trends in Medical Education.   Jonas (1981) described the current status of medical education in the United States as "Disease-Oriented Physician Education" (DOPE) and believes that to achieve the health goals of the United States it will have to change to "Health-Oriented Physician Education" (HOPE) (p. 199).

In September 1986, the Association of Teachers of Preventive Medicine published its first *Directory and Profile of Academic Units in Preventive Medicine,* which listed all United States medical school academic units in preventive medicine that responded to their questionnaire, and profiled information on those academic units. Data were compiled on the activities of 102 of the 127 settings identified as engaging in preventive education. The data indicated that 126 academic units in preventive medicine existed in the United States' 128 medical schools. Sixty-six percent (68) of those responding reported that within the past three years they had a curriculum review or an organizational or curricular change that had an impact on the major teaching activities or other responsibilities of their preventive medicine unit. Fifty-one percent (52) of these stated that the reviews and/or changes had been positive (Association of Teachers of Preventive Medicine, 1986). The growth of the primary care movement has emphasized viewing the person as a whole, has generated more interest in preventive care, and has increased the emphasis on counseling and education. The primary care movement has brought forth the additional medical specialty of family practice, which has defined itself as different from other specialties with its focus on the family and health education. Family practitioners originally designated nurses and health education specialists to be the patient education coordinators (Bartlett, 1984). Family practitioners are discouraged (as are internists and pediatricians) from doing much primary prevention, because it takes a lot of time and is so poorly reimbursed compared to other more specific diagnostic and therapeutic interventions (Relman, 1982).

According to Dr. Joan Altekruse, President of the Association for Teachers of Preventive Medicine, the attitudes of "encouraging numbers" of medical students are beginning to change toward appreciating prevention of disease and seeking educational and practice resources to evaluate the potential of preventive medical care. Altekruse suggests that the knowledge base and workload are present to support an independent specialty practice in preventive medicine (1986, p. 5).

A 1985 study of the preventive care attitudes of medical students revealed that third year medical students expressed a high level of confidence in the ability of physicians to provide immunizations, blood pressure control, cancer detection education, family planning, health counseling/education, and sexually transmitted disease prevention. These students had low confidence in the ability of physicians to provide smoking cessation, nutrition counseling/education, weight reduction, life-style modification, occupational health/safety education, risk factor analysis, genetic counseling, and exercise/physical fitness programs (Scott & Neighbor, 1985).

Louisiana State University (LSU) Medical School introduced a health promotion program for medical students for the 1986–1987 academic year. The purpose of this course was to encourage medical students to learn to take responsibility for their own psycho-social health and well-being early in their medical careers so they would be better able to cope with the stressors they encounter as they continue their education and go into practice. LSU plans to expand the program to all four years of medical school (Wolf & Randall, 1987).

In a 1985 cooperative agreement, the Association of Teachers of Preventive Medicine with the Centers for Disease Control initiated the development of an Inventory of Knowledge and Skills Relating to Disease Prevention and Health Promotion for the purposes of highlighting fundamental concepts, scientific principles, and professional skills all undergraduate medical students should master. The Inventory also offered guidance to medical faculty related to disease prevention and health promotion curriculum content. The plan is for this Inventory to be reviewed and revised periodically to reflect current trends in medical education. It was first published in

December 1986 with the hope that health care educators and practitioners would talk together about future revisions of the Inventory and confirm its utility as a tool to change the way prevention would be taught and practiced (Barbour, 1986). It was hoped that the Inventory would serve as a means to effectively integrate preventive education into medical student and medical resident education (Beasley, 1986).

The Inventory (1987) suggested that a physician's responsibilities in disease prevention and health promotion include "developing productive partnerships with the full range of individuals and groups concerned with disease prevention and health promotion, including other health professionals, official health agencies, private community-based health organizations and the media" (p. 14). The Inventory also identifies patient education and counseling as essential components of clinical practice and identifies the importance of health behavior theory, strategies for modifying harmful health behaviors with the necessary follow-up, continuity, and assessment of care outcomes. The Inventory encourages the development of skills in identifying and using other sources of patient education: hospital personnel, voluntary community agency literature, and programs. The Inventory suggests further that strategies should be developed for the systematic evaluation of the effectiveness and costs of including disease prevention and health promotion content in patient care. As part of this evaluation, quality of life should be considered along with other factors in outcome evaluation (*Inventory*, 1986). Calkins (1987) recognized the Inventory as a "significant achievement," but he stated that its implementation will be a challenge.

Campbell and Valente (1983) have suggested three areas in which additional education for physicians should be provided. The first is in medical school where health education should be considered as basic to the practice of medicine as is clinical training. The second area includes communication and health education/promotion skills provided through postgraduate programs, internships, and residencies. The last suggestion is to provide education using Continuing Medical Education (CME) programs. There are a few states (Maryland being one) that already require physician participation at CME programs for continued licensing. This latter suggestion is addressed by Weinberg and Andrus (1982) as well. They reported that opportunities for physicians to acquire new knowledge and skills in prevention via CME are limited and not growing substantially. CME directors have difficulty finding trained faculty who are willing to present courses on these subjects.

Although progress towards the incorporation of health promotion/disease prevention content into medical education and continuing medical education is evident, it remains slow and continues to meet resistance (Passing Review,

1986). Dr. J. Robert Buchanan (Passing Review, 1986), a plenary session presenter at the 1986 meeting of the Association of American Medical Colleges stated:

> Academic medicine's energy is largely focused on maintaining the "status quo" of our medical school undergraduate curricula and graduate training programs. Our faculty populate the boards and specialty societies that have been so resistant to creating program requirements focused on the changing needs of our society. (p. 53)

Even those physicians who are truly interested in incorporating health promotion/disease prevention activities into their practices face many obstacles. The literature that addresses these obstacles is summarized below.

OBSTACLES CITED BY PRACTICING PHYSICIANS THAT PREVENT THEM FROM INVOLVEMENT WITH HEALTH EDUCATION

The Center for Health Education Inc., located in Baltimore, Maryland, hosted a "Physician Health Education State-of-the-Art Forum" on December 14, 1982 to identify barriers that precluded physicians from being more involved in health education/health promotion and to determine appropriate health education techniques for physicians. These barriers are addressed by this forum, as well as those identified in other literature, are discussed below.

Lack of Time

The obstacle most frequently mentioned by physicians attending the Forum was the lack of time to treat behavioral risks (Campbell & Valente, 1983; Orleans et al., 1985). Regardless of whether this is an attitudinal issue or a real constraint, health education/promotion is easily disregarded with statements about the lack of time available. Health education/promotion *does* take time and energy on the part of the physician and the patient, and many physicians as discouraged from doing much primary prevention because it does take a lot of time . . . compared to more specific diagnostic and therapeutic interventions (Relman, 1982).

Lack of Reimbursement

The second issue identified by physicians attending the Forum was the cost of providing health education without third party reimbursement. Current patterns by third party reimbursers do not encourage physicians to do much more than diagnose and treat a patient and then to move on to the next one (Kernaghan & Giloth, 1983). This barrier has been previously discussed in detail.

Lack of Interest and Pessimism About Outcomes

Physicians place a significant amount of the blame for the obstacles to the incorporation of health promotion/disease prevention efforts into their practice on the programs and the patient. As mentioned previously, clinicians place a relative lack of value on health promotion activities, perhaps because they do not believe they have impacted patients' health by means of preventive approaches as they feel they have with medical treatment (Fleming, 1980). Many physicians question the value of health promotion and the clinical efficacy of some of the programs, such as stress management and fitness (Fletcher, 1985). In the 1985 study by Orleans et al., 50% of responding physicians reported they lacked confidence in the effectiveness of available health behavior change programs. Ford and Ford (1983) reported physicians have the perception that patients are not interested in changing health behaviors, and physicians believe compliance with behavioral advice is low (Orlandi, 1987; Kernaghan & Giloth, 1983).

According to Hankey (1987), the problem with implementing health promotion is "the lack of 'doctor compliance' with published health promotion protocols, and not with patient cooperation" (p. 25). Hankey objects to the word compliance because it denotes a condescending attitude toward the patient—implying that the patient is supposed to do what the doctor says. Hankey believes this is inappropriate when addressing disease prevention and health promotion where it is the patient's philosophy about health and voluntary risk that determines patient behavior.

In a 1985 study of a national sample of 610 family practice physicians, Orleans et al. reported two-thirds of respondents were pessimistic about the abilities of individuals to change behavior. Ford and Ford (1983) reported that 57% of the physicians responding to their study believed that patients themselves were obstacles to the incorporation of health promotion/disease prevention activities into primary care, because of the patients' lack of interest in being taught about health.

Lack of Confidence Due to the Medical Education Process

The inadequacies of the medical education process have been discussed in detail and physicians have reported their awareness of this inadequacy. In one study, 30% of physicians reported their own education was inadequate for treating health behavior problems (Orleans et al., 1985).

Poor Coordination For and Poor Follow Up On Referrals

Another area in which physicians assume some of the blame and also focus some of the blame on the patient is in regard to referrals. In a 1985 study by Orleans et al., two-thirds of the physician respondents noted that their patients resisted referrals to mental health professionals and self-help groups for behavior change. Additionally, 25% of the physicians reported there was poor coordination with referral agencies, and 20% indicated a shortage of available referral sources.

In 1982, McGinnis suggested that one role of physicians was to refer the patient to other health providers or community resources that could supply the necessary services more efficiently and/or at less cost. McGinnis stated that traditional medical education does not prepare physicians to be comfortable as referrers, and that physicians' lack of familiarity with community resources contributes to this difficulty. McNamara (1982) supported the idea of referral, stating that many preventive services do not require the direct services of physicians and may be offered by those better trained and at less expense, such as nurse practitioners and/or health educators.

Dunn (1982) supported this concept as well and stated patients should be referred to other health professionals or self-help groups and that other professionals such as nurses, health educators, and social workers were capable of carrying out health promotion activities that would be more cost effective than extensive personal involvement by physicians. In addition, these services would not necessarily increase physicians' costs (Campbell & Valente, 1983).

Territoriality and Concern About the Patient Self-Care Movement

Closely associated with poor coordination with the referral process is the issue of territoriality among health care providers. The 1984 conference of organizations devoted to implementing strategies for attainment of the 1990 health objectives revealed territorial conflict among primary care health organizations and health professionals, which presented a real threat to the progress of health promotion (USDHSS, 1984b).

Physician reluctance to participate in a situation that has the potential to provide positive outcomes is based on the notion that health education and the self-care movement could conceivably undermine medical power because the educational model promotes individual responsibility. This takes some of the power and paternalism away from the provider. Physicians may believe informing patients about self-care will increase patients' ability to identify deficiencies in medical care and initiate price and product comparison among providers. Self-care could decrease the need for professional intervention, and recognizing health educators as providers decreases medicine's control over the nature of clinical services. As it stands now, the health educator is one of a minority of health professionals who can act without physician permission (the others being optometrists, dentists, and psychologists) (Bartlett & Windsor, 1985).

The participants at the 1984 conference of organizations devoted to implementing strategies for attainment of the 1990 health objectives stated it was apparent that many health professionals did not have adequate education to plan, implement, and evaluate health promotion programs (USDHHS, 1984b). Many health care providers do not understand the relationship between individual life-style and its effects on health, and many health care providers are threatened by the idea of patient self-care and consumer responsibility for their own health decisions. Health care providers believe they will lose clinical power and authority and will take in less money if consumers become self-care proponents (Green, 1985), or if consumers are referred to other categories of health care providers. Most physicians want to control all aspects of patient care that traditionally have been considered within the realm of the practice of medicine. Physicians are reluctant to delegate part of a patient's care or to share the care with another person. The responsibility for physicians to direct patient care is instilled in medical school. While physicians have been comfortable letting some professionals become involved with patient care, such as nurses, therapists, and pharmacists, they have allowed this only because these professions have a long history of hospital practice and what they do is visible, understandable, and under the jurisdiction of the physicians. Educators are the newest members of the team and cannot claim a past record. Until physicians recognize the right and the competence of the health educator, the services offered by health educators will be suspect, *particularly* if they are seen as in competition with physicians' own private practice (Kernaghan & Giloth, 1983). The 1984 conference of organizations devoted to implementing strategies for attainment of the 1990 health objectives proposed a multidisciplinary approach to meeting the health promotion/disease prevention needs of patients because the complexity of the field of health education requires the expertise of a variety of health professionals such as health educators, psychologists, behavioral scientists, nurses, physicians, dietitians, and communication experts (USDHHS, 1984b).

Additional Barriers

Additional barriers discussed at the Center for Health Education forum was the belief held by some physicians that health education was not their responsibility, whereas other physicians believed they were offering some form of health education whenever they prescribed a medical regimen. The question of ethics was another issue raised by some of the physicians who asked if it was ethical for a physician or anyone to attempt to change the behavior of another person. The counterargument is: Would it be unethical *not* to attempt to change unhealthy habits or behaviors (Campbell & Valente, 1983)? Twenty-five percent of the respondents in the 1985 study by Orleans et al. believed that health promotion activities were inappropriate because "life-style is a matter of personal choice" (p. 641).

The last obstacles to physician involvement with health education in their practice identified by Forum participants related to competition from negative influences and lack of good materials to support health education efforts. Advertising, movies, television, and radio programs tend to encourage unhealthy habits such as smoking, alcohol consumption, and eating of salty and high sugar content foods. At the same time that these inappropriate behaviors are encouraged by the media, the media also show that physicians and medicine can cure most ills, thus eliminating the incentive for the patient to take responsibility (Campbell & Valente, 1983; USDHHS, 1984b).

These concerns suggest a need for a collaborative agreement between physicians and health educators in which each professions' services augment those of the other, rather than one replacing the other. Each is allowed to do what they have been educated to do best and enjoy most, with the ultimate outcome being improved patient care and improved patient satisfaction.

A recent statement by the American Heart Association suggested that technological advances in medicine over the next four years will be overshadowed by the emphasis on preventive medicine, health education, and more basic approaches to health maintenance. It was also predicted that nonphysicians will provide more health care in the future (Passing Review, 1987). "The time is ripe for ever-enhanced collaboration between the primary care and prevention communities" (Fried, 1987, p. 9). In 1985, Scott and Neighbor suggested that if some aspects of preventive care services were not suited to medical practice, collaboration with health care providers from other professions could be fostered. In 1983, Ford and Ford asked physicians who they thought was suitable to assume the primary responsibility for health education. Physicians, professional health educators, and public health personnel received the most first preference. Eighty-one percent thought efforts should be directed at children and young adults. Although these physician respondents thought that physicians should have the primary responsibility for health education, they believed most have little interest in teaching basic health principles.

In summary, it appears that at least at the present time, reliance on physicians to provide the bulk of health education is unwise. Many physicians question whether or not they have the skills necessary to educate patients about life-style changes, they lack the confidence and the time to encourage the behavior changes that would affect life habits (Campbell & Valente, 1983; Kaplan, 1985), medical education does not appear to be incorporating prevention experiences at a fast enough rate, and even if this situation were improved, physicians also doubt their patients would heed their suggestions regarding behavioral change (Haynes, 1979). Furthermore, physicians are not reimbursed for providing health promotion/disease prevention education.

ATTITUDES OF HEALTH ORGANIZATIONS AND GROUPS TOWARD HEALTH EDUCATION

The attitudes towards health promotion/disease prevention held by physicians, health care consumers, the American Medical Association (AMA), and health insurance agencies have a significant impact on the present and future incorporation of health education into primary care practice settings. This section addresses the attitudes of each of these groups towards health promotion/disease prevention activities.

Attitudes of Physicians Toward Involvement in Health Education

Even though some reports indicated that preventive medicine is seen as peripheral to the central body of medical practice (Relman, 1982), it is important to know what importance physicians do attach to health promotion behaviors. In this way, one can identify those aspects that can be emphasized in communicating with physicians regarding the information they may provide to their patients. Boynton (1986) compared the self-reported personal health risk behaviors of 119 medical faculty with 136 nonmedical faculty and 330 medical students. Faculty physicians consumed significantly more wine, hard liquor, and mood-altering or relaxant drugs than nonmedical faculty; and physician faculty reported significant differences in alcohol consumption, overweight, and smoking risk behaviors over medical students. These findings suggested that faculty physicians were not acting as exemplary role models of health promotion behaviors.

A 1981 survey of slightly less than 500 Massachusetts primary care physicians reported physician support for the importance of healthy behaviors such as not smoking cigarettes, avoiding excess calories, and using a seat belt. Of the 26 behaviors listed on the questionnaire, there was a significant difference found among the attitudes of the general and family practice physicians and internists. The authors found that general practitioners, the group with the highest mean age, gathered behavioral information from their patients significantly less often than their younger colleagues. This 1981 Massachusetts survey of primary care physicians did not include specific measures about promotion of risk reduction and life-style modification, but 81% of the respondents reported they personally provided patient education rather than relying on a nurse or other health professional (Wechsler, Levin, & Idelson, 1983). In view of the average length of an office visit (11 minutes for primary care physicians and 18 minutes for internists) (Mendenhall, 1981), it appears that not much time can be spent actually addressing health promotion/disease prevention concerns. In the Wechsler study, physicians were asked how well prepared they considered themselves in helping patients achieve behavior changes. Although they felt qualified to counsel patients regarding smoking (58%), they expressed less confidence in counseling about the use of alcohol, exercise, diet, drugs, and stress. The latter behaviors are listed in descending order with only 29% of the respondents feeling prepared to counsel about stress. In response to questions regarding their success in helping patients change their behavior, 43% of the physicians believed they were at least *somewhat successful* in helping patients to change, and only 3% to 8% thought that they were *very successful* in helping patients change their behavior (Wechsler et al., 1983). In another study of 230 primary care physicians in Florida, there was widespread belief that health education was an effective means of altering behavior and yet, again, only 3% to 8% of the respondents considered their own teaching and counseling regarding health promotion to be very successful in changing their patients' behaviors (Ford & Ford, 1983).

Physicians surveyed by Logsdon and Rosen (1984) expressed interest in providing more preventive care and 92% agreed they should spend more time on preventive patient services. Sobal, Valente, Muncie, Levine, & Deforge (1985) surveyed 1,715 primary care physicians in the state of Maryland and reported a consensus across specialties: health behaviors were rated as very important. Fifteen health behaviors were considered very important for promoting the health of the average person. These health behaviors are listed below in descending order by percentage of physicians considering the health behavior to be very important: Eliminate cigarette smoking, 94%; protective equipment/clothing around harmful substances, 82%; avoid excess caloric intake, 73%; eat a balanced diet, 68%; always use seat belts, 67%; knowledge about drug contents, 59%; avoid unnecessary x-rays, 52%; avoid saturated fat foods, 52%; drink alcohol moderately, 52%; eliminate cigar smoking, 43%; avoid undue stress, 42%; decrease salt consumption, 41%; avoid high cholesterol foods, 41%; eliminate pipe smoking, 40%; eat breakfast every morning, 33%; get 7 hours sleep each night, 30%; annual physical examination, 28%; aerobic activity 3 times/week, 27%; limit daily caffeine intake, 23%; practice relaxation methods, 20%; minimize sugar intake, 15%; drink no alcohol at all, 15%; baseline exercise test 12%; annual exercise test, 6%; and take vitamin supplements, 6%.

On the other hand, Nutting (1986) reported that physicians perceived health promotion to be the narrow perspective of immunizations, screening for asymptomatic disease, and informing and advising patients rather than taking a more active role to promote behavioral change. Some physicians believe that health promotion is uninteresting and professionally unrewarding compared to their roles as healers and alleviators of human suffering (Fleming, 1980; Nutting, 1986). "The rewards of prevention are much less striking and immediate than those of curative medicine" (Weinberg & Andrus, 1982, p. 213). Orleans et al., (1985) reported that when primary care physicians do intervene, they apply health education techniques that are ineffective when used alone to alter habits and behavior, they rarely if ever apply effective newly developed behavior change strategies, and they have very little confidence in their ability to help patients change health behaviors. Primary care physicians' pessimism is based on repeated failures to see their patients lose weight, quit smoking, or increase their exercise. Many physicians lack the training and support services to provide health promotion, and many physicians are poorly informed about effective community-based health promotion programs.

ATTITUDES OF PRIMARY CARE MEDICAL SPECIALTY GROUPS TOWARD INVOLVEMENT IN HEALTH EDUCATION

Because the preventive illness literature is filled with studies such as those cited above, many authors have concluded that physicians are uninterested in prevention. However, a 1987 report by Robert Fried concluded that organized medicine, and particularly all primary care specialties, have very quickly become involved in implementing clinical preventive services. Family medicine has taken the lead and offers the single best hope for health promotion (Nutting, 1986). Family medicine's goal is to provide comprehensive and preventive care to their patients (Kottke, Foels, Hill, Choi, & Fenderson, 1983). Many physician organizations are encouraging their members to assume greater roles in teaching and counseling (Kernaghan & Giloth, 1983). The American Academy of Family Physicians, currently focusing on a major smoking cessation effort, has formally recognized patient education as having a positive effect on the health of patients and as helping to control costs by preventing catastrophic episodes of illness and by minimizing the debilitating effects of chronic disease (Kernaghan & Giloth, 1983). At the October 1986 meeting of the American Academy of Family Physicians a presentation entitled "The Family Physician as Health Promotion Specialist" was offered (Fried, 1987).

Other efforts by major medical specialty organizations were reported by Fried in 1987. These include the Society of Teachers of Family Medicine, which has established a Working Group or Health Promotion and Disease Prevention and has added several health promotion textbooks to its official book list. The American College of Physicians has developed prevention reviews and is looking for means to expand its educational efforts on the value of preventive medicine to consumers as well as its members. The American College of Obstetricians and Gynecologists (ACOG) has a long history of interest in prevention. ACOG has established scientific panels to explore preventive measures of particular relevance to females such as cancer screening, osteoporosis prevention, and prevention of teenage pregnancy (Fried, 1987). Obstetricians and gynecologists have assumed responsibility for maintaining and promoting the health of women throughout their reproductive years, to provide the best possible environment for the birth and rearing of healthy children. ACOG recognizes the value of community preventive services to respond to teenage pregnancy, low birthweight babies, and one of the higher infant mortality rates among developed nations (Coffelt, 1987).

Logsdon and Rosen (1984) reported that physicians have recognized a need and have been providing patient education for a number of years. However, these patient education programs are oriented to illnesses, such as diabetes management, rather than disease prevention or health promotion (Logsdon & Rosen, 1984). However, even with these efforts, physicians still fail to provide the recommended preventive care to their patients (Calkins, 1987). Earlier it was reported that a national sample of 610 family practice physicians indicated 40% of their patients smoked, 40% were significantly overweight, and close to 70% did not pursue adequate exercise (Orleans et al., 1985). Another study showed that only 52% of internists reported counseling more than 75% of smokers to reduce or stop smoking, and only 15% of internists reported they counseled more than 75% of their patients who did not exercise to start a regular exercise program (Wells, Lewis, Leake, Schleiter, & Brook, 1986).

Attitudes of Health Care Consumers/Patients Toward Health Education

In spite of widespread dissatisfaction with the status of health care in the United States, consumers continue to perceive their primary care-giver, the physician, as their best source of health information (David & Boldt, 1980; Kernaghan & Giloth, 1983; Nutting, 1986; Rimer et al., 1986). At the same time, however, patients/consumers reported a perceived relative lack of advice regarding health behavior (Clearie, Blair, & Ward, 1982), infrequently reported their physician as a source of encouragement to change health related behaviors (USDHEW, 1979), and saw preventive medicine as peripheral to the core of medical practice (Relman, 1982).

Regarding the status of the population, a recent publication of the National Center for Health Statistics revealed from interviews with 170,302 adults from age 18 to over 65 years of age that 45% considered themselves overweight; 37% were trying to lose weight; 82% were eating fewer calories to try to lose weight; 66% stated that their health care provider rarely if ever discussed eating proper foods; for 37% of the women it had been two or more years since they had last had a Pap test; for 51% of the women it had been over a year since a health care provider had examined their breasts; and 66% examined their breasts less than 6 times per year (which included 26% who stated they had never examined their own breasts); 52% of the respondents felt that they were under moderate to severe amounts of stress; 41% stated they exercised or played sports regularly; 30% smoked; and 28% were moderate to heavy consumers of alcoholic beverages (United States Department of Health and Human Services, 1985).

Yoder et al. (1985) studied a convenience sample of 104 patients awaiting treatment in a midwest emergency department to determine health attitudes of patients in this setting. The authors' found those patients who perceived that an illness would be more serious if contracted were more apt to practice disease prevention behaviors. Although most of these subjects (92%) expressed belief in the value of health behaviors one could adopt by oneself, the number of those who actually practiced disease prevention behaviors was less (69%). Study participants who practiced health behaviors were the ones who expressed belief in their efficacy for achieving and maintaining good health, but the practice of these disease prevention behaviors was not associated with health beliefs. Eighty-three percent of respondents practiced disease prevention regardless of their health beliefs, particularly those who thought the disease would be serious if they contracted it. The authors interpreted this finding to mean that patients believe going to the doctor somehow prevents the occurrence of disease (Yoder et al., 1985). The authors also found that as individuals aged, they reported themselves engaging in less disease prevention behavior. Two reasons were suggested by the authors to explain this behavior. The first explanation was that older people may be resigned to the inevitability of disease and therefore no longer see any value in disease prevention behaviors. The second reason was that the older population had avoided serious disease for many years and therefore perceived themselves as less vulnerable. Some of the respondents reported it was silly to go to the doctor if there was nothing wrong with a person's health (Yoder et al., 1985).

Attitudes of consumers toward the health promotion efforts of their physicians were reflected in the results of a 1979 poll in which 57% of the respondents said they could be significantly helped to eat a healthy diet if it was recommended by their doctor, while only 16% of those eating a special diet were prompted to do so by their doctor's advice. Seventy percent of the respondents said information from their doctor would be useful and reliable, but only 47% reported they currently received a lot of information about health and medical care from their doctor (Logsdon, 1982).

Fletcher (1985) believes the attitudes of consumers needs to change. Patients do not usually think of visiting their physician for health promotion services and many are reluctant to spend money on wellness care. Many consumers are not willing to make the time and energy commitment nor the self-sacrifices needed to achieve life-style changes. It is a lot easier if the physician could just prescribe a pill for them rather than the consumer making changes in behavior (Fletcher, 1985).

Attitudes of the American Medical Association Toward Health Education

The American Medical Association (AMA) is the largest American organization of physicians and recognizes the important relationship between health information and health management. In a 1979 statement about patient education, the American Medical Association's House of Delegates reported that the physician and the patient share in the continuous responsibility to participate in patient education services, which are designed to help the family and the patient effectively manage their health (Kernaghan & Giloth, 1983; Squyres, 1985).

In 1980, the AMA resolved to increase its activity in the promotion of health education in schools and physicians' offices (Mullen & Katayama, 1985). In 1983, the Council on Scientific Affairs of the American Medical Association published a recommendation on medical evaluations of healthy persons, which included periodic evaluations based on age and sex of the patient and encouraged patient education for prevention. This was the first report addressing medical evaluations of healthy persons to be issued since 1947 (Logsdon & Rosen, 1984).

More recently, the Director of the Health Education Unit at the AMA noted that health education is now a concern of physicians. He indicated that there has been a steady increase in enthusiasm for patient education and health promotion. The AMA has established a competetive action plan offered to member physicians suggesting the use of health promotion as a marketing tool to gain an advantage over their competitors in an increasingly competitive market (Mullen & Katayama, 1985).

Attitudes of the American Hospital Association Toward Health Education

Since the 1960s, the same social and economic factors that brought the concepts and practice of health promotion into public view have generated interest in health promotion activities by hospitals. Hospitals have expanded their traditional patient education efforts into community health education and employee health programs. For these programs to be utilized effectively, physician support and involvement is essential (Kernaghan & Gilroth, 1983).

The American Hospital Association believes that patient education services should enable individuals and families to make informed decisions about their health, to manage their illnesses, and to implement follow-up care at home. Hospitals identified the target population as those individuals who were awaiting and/or undergoing medical treatment in institutions and in physicians' offices (Squyres, 1985).

Attitudes of Health Insurance Agencies Toward Health Education

Traditionally health insurance benefits have not included preventive services. The basic purpose of health insurance has been to protect people from economic losses related to unanticipated, expensive illness. Because preventive care is not unanticipated nor expensive when compared to hospitalization, it has usually been excluded from health insurance policies. Other reasons cited by the health insurance agencies for not reimbursing preventive services included a lack of demand (Riedel & Gibbs, 1987); claims that the reimbursement already provided should include health education activities (Campbell & Valente, 1983), that illness preventive services that were not illness related and were usually excluded, and that preventive care was a budgetable expense that the insured person should be expected to pay (Logsdon & Rosen, 1984). The only preventive care covered by Medicare was the pneumococcal vaccine, and Blue Cross-Blue Shield coverage generally has been limited to hospital-based inpatient education services (Logsdon et al., 1982). In Logsdon and Rosen's (1984) study, it was found that 30% of adults and 23% of children were covered by their insurance policies for preventive services. At the same time, 87% of patients were either very or somewhat interested in preventive services being covered by their health insurance and were willing to pay from $5.00 to $25.00 per month for preventive coverage.

Health insurance agencies expressed concern that not enough research had been done to show the effectiveness and cost benefits of health education. However, it was also suggested that improvements in communication, changes in the physician/patient relationship, and better coordination with support groups and facilities would not necessarily increase physicians' costs. In fact, in some cases, costs may be reduced and income increased by elimination of problems such as broken appointments (Campbell & Valente, 1983).

With the dramatic rise in health care costs, the predominant concern for third party payers is cost containment. In an effort to control health care costs, the health insurance industry and employers have tried cost sharing, higher deductibles and co-insurance, second surgical opinions, and worksite wellness programs. Additionally, some have decreased health insurance benefits and/or eliminated new benefits. Until preventive care can be proven cost effective, it is unlikely preventive coverage will be included in programs (Logsdon and Rosen, 1984).

The Office of Disease Prevention and Health Promotion (ODPHP) is currently undertaking a study with the Hospital Insurance Association of American to examine preferred provider organization's (PPO) offering of preventive services. As a result of this study ODPHP hopes to initiate coverage of preventive services and effective preventive services benefit plans (Harrell, 1986).

A 1987 report of the Blue Cross and Blue Shield Organization noted that their 78 nonprofit plans provided health insurance to one-third of the population of the United States and that the majority of the plans provided disease prevention and health promotion coverage to subscribers. These plans incorporated preventive care benefits such as adult immunizations, periodic physical examinations, and/or well-child benefits as part of the traditional fee-for-service coverage. Thirty plans provided health promotion programs (most often worksite health promotion programs) to their accounts, which may include needs assessment, health risk interventions, and program evaluation. Ten plans offered some type of life-style premium rating such as nonsmoker premium discounts. It was predicted that disease prevention/health promotion benefits will continue to develop in the plans because of the competition from prevention oriented organizations such as HMOs, the needs and demands of the accounts, and the "good sense of programs that help prevent disease and promote health" (Riedel & Gibbs, 1987, p. 23).

SETTINGS FOR PATIENT EDUCATION

Currently health education takes place in a variety of different patient care settings with varying degrees of interest, effort, success, and support. These settings include health maintenance organizations (HMOs), hospitals, primary care, private practice settings, and physician group practice settings.

Health Maintenance Organizations

Health Maintenance Organizations (HMOs) provide for prepaid health plans, which include office visits, lab tests, hospitalizations, and health promotion activities for one fixed monthly or biweekly fee (Cohn, 1985). HMOs began as co-op programs during the 1930s when a few dissatisfied consumers and some independent-minded physicians joined forces. This concept was fought by the AMA, with local medical societies (who control hospital staffs) refusing hospital privileges to HMO doctors. The AMA called it "corporate medicine" and believed that salaried doctors, managed by non-doctors, would destroy the doctor-patient relationship. Throughout the 1930s and 1940s, the concept was fought by the AMA. Only after a series of federal criminal indictments, many trials, and a conviction for restraint of trade were physicians who were employed by the HMOs allowed to admit patients to hospitals (Cohn, 1985, p. 14).

The actual name for health maintenance organizations was not coined until the 1970s when President Nixon supported the concept of engaging doctors to provide health care for a flat payment. The support came as a result of the increasing costs of health care. The prepaid plans generally only hospitalized their members when absolutely necessary, and they discharged them as soon as possible (Cohn, 1985). HMO physicians were usually housed under one roof and had their own hospital facility. Health insurance designed to promote health rather than illness was evident in health maintenance organizations. The more people remained healthy and did not need to use this prepaid health care delivery system, the more money could be made by the system. Some HMOs emphasized health education/promotion services (Polakoff, 1982; USDHHS, 1984b), prevention, and self-care, at least in principle; and this prepayment type of insurance plan became a competitor of the traditional fee-for-service nature of other insurance plans (Green, 1985).

Current literature indicates less health promotion activity in HMOs than expected, primarily based on the lack of clear evidence of the impact on morbidity and mortality coupled with the time lag between health promotion activities and projected onset of the illness that has been prevented (Nutting, 1986). Dunn (1982) cited efforts to hold down utilization rates as having reduced the opportunities for educating enrollees in health promotion/disease prevention behaviors.

Prevention programs are the last to be adopted into a health service and are the first to go when finances are no longer free flowing. This is true of HMOs as well. Faust (1986) cited four impediments to providing prevention services in the HMO setting. The first was competition, which forced premiums down and thereby pressured the organization to decrease expenses. The second was the lack of understanding of the value of preventive services on the part of the general population. The third was the lack of data indicating that economic benefits of prevention services were equal to costs. The fourth was the disease orientation of providers. Lastly, the rapid turnover in many HMO memberships meant that the benefits of their health promotion efforts may not have been realized while the enrollee was still a member of their organization.

Fee-for-service doctors began to respond to HMOs by organizing into a concept of "HMOs without walls," called Independent Practice Associations (IPAs). These groups of doctors (sometimes as many as 1,000 and more) provided much the same package as the HMOs, but they continued to practice in their own offices. An additional spin-off in the competitive market was the preferred provider organization (PPO), which typically provided all care for a flat monthly charge if the member used the plan's "preferred" hospital and the plan's "preferred" doctors. If the member chose to go elsewhere, all of the bill might not be paid (Cohn, 1985). Patient education in IPAs and PPOs has not been adequately addressed in the literature.

Hospitals

Because hospitals were viewed by the public as centers for health information, it was to their advantage to offer patient education programs and to have their employed health professionals act as role models for positive health behaviors. Many hospitals have taken a leadership role in providing appropriate health information and education to their communities and their employees (Squyres, 1985).

During the last ten years, hospitals have become increasingly interested in developing health education/promotion programs for their communities. A 1979 study by the American Hospital Association reported that 50% of the 5,663 responding hospitals revealed the existence of this type of program. The more successful of these programs were in large teaching hospitals and employed four or more full-time community health education specialists (USDHHS, 1984b).

Primary Care Private Practice

Most Americans receive their regular medical care from primary care providers (National Center for Health Statistics, 1980). Primary care is defined as first-contact care that is comprehensive and continuous (Nutting, 1986). The primary care setting was considered fertile ground for health promotion activities as the physician followed the patient over time; was generally trusted by the patient; and, while referring the patient to specialists in specific areas as the need arose, usually maintained responsibility for the patient (Nutting, 1986). Primary care physicians have the most contacts with the healthy population, particularly children and young adults. Consequently, these physicians have the greatest opportunity to help patients avoid future problems (McNamara, 1982). In 1984, Americans made an estimated 400 million visits annually to physicians' offices for primary care (Mullen and Katayama, 1985). This is a large number of people who could be readily reached by health promotion/disease prevention efforts. In 1981, approximately 286,500 nonfederal physicians in the United States were seeing patients in their offices. The primary care specialties made up 45% of these office-based physicians: pediatrics, 6%; internal medicine, 15%; obstetrics and gynecology, 7%; and family and general practice, 17% (AMA, 1983).

Mendenhall (1981) reported the average length of visits to primary care physicians (other than internists) was approximately 11 minutes. Internists, who were more likely to see sicker patients have an average visit length of 18 minutes. Orleans et al. (1985) reported from their national sample of 610 family practice physicians that family practice physicians treat an average of 34.2 patients a day. Kehrer, Sloan, and Woolridge (1984) reported from a national telephone survey of office-based primary care physicians in 1979, that primary care physicians see an average of 109 patients per week with a range of 19–22 minutes per visit. Ford and Ford (1983) reported that primary care physicians responding to their survey saw an average of 133 patients/week. The percentage of encounters involving well patients were: General Practice—16.3%, Family Practice—10.3%, Pediatrics—25.9%, Internal Medicine—6.6%, and Obstetrics/Gynecology—43.1% (Mendenhall, 1981).

Until recently, relatively little was known about the extent to which primary care physicians and members of their office staffs engaged in health-promotion education and counseling with their patients. What was known suggested that educational interventions to reduce risk and promote health varied widely and were inconsistent in both quantity and quality (Mullen & Katayama, 1985). A 1986 report of recently graduated internists revealed they rely almost exclusively on face-to-face contact for counseling about smoking and exercise. Ninety percent of responding internists indicated they discussed the risks and benefits of changing health-related behavior and suggested specific steps; 66% explored the patient's feelings about the habit. Of those who did counsel about the habit, 8%–15% did so at the initial visit, 57%–61% counseled less than two minutes per visit, and 36%–47% initiated counseling only when the habit presented an immediate health hazard. Often the counseling was related to complications about having smoked or not exercised. Only 15% stated they counseled most of their patients with poor exercise habits about regular exercise, whereas 56% counseled most of their patients with already established heart disease about exercise (Wells et al., 1986). In general, the internists were less likely to counsel about exercise than about smoking. This may be due to the fact that the evidence linking smoking to cardiovascular disease risk (and the risk of other illness) is clearer than that for regular exercise (Wells et al., 1986).

Mendenhall (1981) described a few indicators of the extent of health-promotion activities compared with other therapeutic procedures: diet and/or exercise were prescribed in only 3%–7% of the ambulatory encounters for primary care physicians; patient counseling, including education of those with chronic conditions, was noted in 12%–20% of visits; drugs (at least one) were prescribed in 27% of visits to obstetricians/gynecologists and 43%–56% of the time for other primary care physicians. The focus, then, remained on medical/pharmacologic interventions.

The health professionals work group of the 1984 conference identified the isolation of private practice as being a problem in the provision of health promotion services (USDHHS, 1984b). Physicians in private practice make the decisions about health promotion alone, if only by default, and usually they are the implementors (Mullen & Katayama, 1985). In organized health care settings (e.g., health maintenance organizations, community clinics, and hospitals) economics may allow health-promotion services to be conducted by appropriately educated staff, thereby relieving physicians from having to take an active role in health promotion (Mullen & Katayama, 1985).

Group Practice

In 1975, 60% of office visits were conducted by physicians in solo practice. This form of practice continues to decline as the trend toward group practice has continued (Mullen & Katayama, 1985). Physician group practices have been evident in the United States for 40 years. Many are small organizations of three to five physicians; some form corporations of large single specialty or multispecialty groups. These group practices open up the possibilities for shared services and group education (Mullen & Katayama, 1985). Patient education programs have been evident in these settings in which the clinical encounter with illness provides the opportunity and time for health education. The physical setting permits cost-sharing of health educators by physicians (USDHHS, 1984b). However, patient education programs in group practice clinics have been oriented to illnesses, such as diabetes management, rather than disease prevention and health promotion (Logsdon & Rosen, 1984). Obstacles to health education in this setting include the reluctance of physicians to use nonphysician health educators, the lack of outside educational materials, the obstacles previously discussed regarding the referral process, and the lack of third party payment for health education (USDHHS, 1984b).

CURRENT HEALTH EDUCATION EFFORTS IN PRIMARY CARE SETTINGS

In the early 1980s, in an effort to meet the 1990 Objectives for the Nation, it was suggested the Department of Health and Human Services (DHHS), and specifically the Public Health Service (PHS), should: support research and evaluation of efforts to develop effective strategies for individual and community behavior change; encourage private foundations and voluntary organizations to help develop health promotion programs for use in health care settings; fund demonstration projects aimed at overcoming barriers to health care provider involvement in health promotion; and use health promotion programs, as appropriate, to develop a competitive edge in the marketplace. Additionally, it was recommended that organizations of the health professions should develop a task force to create a cooperative and coordinated approach to health promotion (USDHHS, 1984b).

A variety of mechanisms for promoting and supporting disease prevention and health promotion efforts in primary care settings are currently being implemented. Some advocate changes in medical education curricula, as discussed earlier in this chapter; others advocate supplementing the physicians with materials; some encourage further education of physicians, and/or the incorporation of other health care providers to provide patient education in the practice. Thus far no qualitative data from evaluations of these efforts is available documenting the effectiveness and efficiency of any of these approaches. The various approaches as identified in the literature are presented in this section.

Concerted efforts in the area of health promotion/disease prevention became more apparent after *Healthy People* (USDHEW, 1979) identified the need for age-specific preventive procedures for patient care. Age-specific preventive procedures were suggested as a replacement for the annual medical examination. *Healthy People* asked for a new commitment to preventive services through disease prevention and health promotion. The age-specific preventive procedures for patient care incorporated clinical and epidemiologic criteria to identify goals and services for nine age groups (newborn through geriatrics and a separate category for pregnancy) to replace the annual medical examination. Specified around these nine groups were preventive services, which included health histories, medical examination procedures, clinical laboratory tests, and patient counseling (Logsdon et al., 1982).

The first and one of the most ambitious and well planned efforts for incorporating health promotion/disease prevention into primary care settings was through the INSURE project. This was a nonprofit, tax-exempt organization developed to conduct a three-year research effort studying health promotion and disease prevention in primary medical care. Specifically, the project was designed to determine the feasibility of implementing preventive services into primary medical care (within multispecialty group practices) as a health insurance benefit, and to assess the short-term impact of this implementation on providers and consumers as well as the long-term impact on cost containment. The program was based on the philosophy that early detection of disease and health promotion among the well and asymptomatic patient could best be accomplished through the primary care physician using a life cycle perspective (Logsdon and Rosen, 1984). A quasi-experimental approach used three study (experimental) group practice sites matched with three control group practice sites at various locations around the United States. At the experimental sites, physicians participated in orientation sessions on recommended preventive services and patient education procedures. Patients were also studied at these sites. The experimental and control group physicians and patients were surveyed before and after the program of intervention was conducted to assess and compare their knowledge, attitudes, and behavior toward health behavior practices (Logsdon et al., 1982). Protocols and educational materials were developed for the participating primary care physicians (general practitioners, internists, obstetrician-gynecologists, pediatricians, and family practitioners). Payments were made to the group practice centers by the INSURE Project, based on an agreed upon payment schedule, with no charge to the study patients. The project team worked with the physicians to assist them in incorporating the life cycle approach with selected patients according to the study protocols. In addition to the age-specific health history, physical exam, clinical laboratory tests, x-ray procedures, and immunizations, 15 minutes of patient education on risk reduction was recommended (Logsdon and Rosen, 1984).

The objectives of the INSURE feasibility study were:

1. To define a life cycle model for age-specific preventive health services including patient education on risk reduction for patients of all ages, and to implement this model at selected study sites by obtaining the participation of primary care physicians in group practice.

2. To develop supporting protocols and educational materials for physicians to use with their patients regarding health promotion in primary medical care.

3. To evaluate, by means of a quasi-experimental research design, the short-term effects of the intervention on physicians and patients (Logsdon & Rosen, 1984, p. 47).

The primary areas of evaluation were to determine the extent to which physicians would be willing to offer and incorporate these services into their practices and the degree to which patients would be willing to use these services. In a study of 1,463 physicians, 92% believed that physicians should incorporate preventive health care into their practices, but 67% stated that one of the major obstacles to practicing preventive care was the lack of insurance reimbursement (Logsdon & Rosen, 1984). Initial results from the INSURE project indicated that interest among respondents to receive this preventive coverage was 87%. When asked how much they would pay for these services, 57% said they would pay $5.00 a month, 9.2% said that they would be willing to pay $15.00 a month, and 2.7% said that they would be willing to pay $25.00 a month. Of the total sample of physicians (1,463), 92% said that physicians should spend more time on preventive services (Logsdon & Rosen, 1984).

The preliminary findings of the INSURE Project indicated that costs (charges) can be controlled if benefits and payment schedules are defined in advance by the providers. Additionally, the short-term effects of this project were encouraging regarding improved health-related behavior changes (e.g., smoking cessation, increased exercise, use of seat belts, and breast self-examinations). The preliminary evidence was encouraging and indicated that with appropriate economic incentives, health promotion services could be provided in primary care settings (Nutting, 1986). The INSURE Project intends to address the behavior changes further in its longitudinal prospective study (Logsdon & Rosen, 1984).

There are other less well-known strategies for incorporating health promotion/disease prevention into primary care settings as well. Prather (1984) and Schneider (1984) have suggested the importance of health education and self-care in two different primary care settings. Prather (1984) reported the importance of patient education in a private obstetric/gynecology practice to transmit accurate health information to clientele who were being bombarded with new information from the media. Prather encouraged physicians to become educators as well as renderers of medical services and to form partnerships with patients. According to Prather, this approach should decrease litigation due to more reasonable expectations on the part of the patient with increased participation and shared responsibility.

Schneider (1984) described the Idaho Wellness Center, a family practice organization with a strong commitment to self-care, based on the belief that the more involved patients become in their care and the more responsibility they assume for their health, the better medical care they will receive. The Center also believed physicians could relate better to those who want to be responsible for their health and to learn how to take care of themselves. Schneider reported satisfaction from practicing with this philosophy, and indicated it has attracted new patient groups to the practice.

Educational efforts and education materials have been another mechanism used to facilitate the implementation of health education into primary care settings. The American Academy of Family Practice has developed an education program on health promotion entitled, Health Education Lifetime Plan. This program plans to provide family practice physicians with factual information on selected topics in preventive medicine, suggestions for managing their practices, reproducible materials for educating their patients, and eventually a newsletter that would be the major vehicle for communication with family practice physicians (Mullen & Katayama, 1985).

In 1981, an innovative program called the Preventive Care Learning Center (PCLC) was established in central Florida to provide family practice residents with a model resource center to enable them to develop patient education or preventive medicine programs and skills to suit personal practice needs. The PCLC serves 5,000 patients/consumers a year and provides patients with a resource center (called the Family Health Center) to help them understand their disease condition and identify life-style changes to help in treatment, prevention, and increased wellness. The PCLC is staffed by health counselors, including a preventive care specialist, a health education specialist (part-time), and a nurse health educator. Referrals to the center are made by the physician who completes a health education prescription. Learning modules use a variety of media; videoplayers, filmstrips, slide/tape players, and programs have been purchased or developed for 30 topic areas. In addition, written materials and body organ models are available for patient and practitioner use (Vartabedian & Hamilton, 1982).

Fletcher (1985) reports on two additional health promotion efforts. The first, the Health-Styles project in Houston, is directed to family practice residents for teaching health promotion skills. The second, Mercy Medical Center in Denver, has developed a 24-module program in health promotion/disease prevention for family practice residents. These modules will eventually be available to all practitioners.

The Center for Health Education (CHE) in Maryland is a physician-based, health promotion assistance project established in 1982 by the Medical and Chirurgical Faculty of the State of Maryland (Med-Chi), which is the State Medical Society, and Blue Cross and Blue Shield of Maryland. CHE is the only state-wide venture of its kind. It is based on the belief that successful health education can have a positive impact on health service utilization. The executive director is a health educator who works with physicians in taking the initiative to encourage and assist their physician colleagues to increase the health education/promotion services offered in their offices and to improve communication skills with their patients (CHE, 1983).

The Society of Teachers of Family Medicine (STFM) has recently formed a Working Group on Health Promotion/Disease Prevention to encourage family medicine programs to develop curricula in health promotion for medical students, residents, faculty, and other health care providers (Passing, 1986). The 1987 annual meeting of the STFM included a full day of seminars and a workshop on the subject of health promotion/disease prevention (Passing, 1987).

SUMMARY

Physicians have the means to shape the course of health promotion efforts depending on whether they decide to leave these activities entirely to others, work in partnership with others, or lay claim to the entire area. What physicians decide will significantly impact on the national health promotion effort.

As Fletcher (1985) suggested:

> Health promotion is not just handing out pamphlets; it takes time, enthusiasm, faith, and the willingness to wait for small, incremental positive changes. Health promotion, which is in its infancy, has a rapidly expanding data base, crosses many clinical disciplines, and is vulnerable to hype and quackery. Unless physicians assume a leadership role in health promotion and act as educators and exemplars, the field of health promotion will be ripe for charlatans. (p. 310)

A number of authors support the concept of a partnership or joint effort among physicians, health educators, and patients to meet the health promotion/disease prevention needs of primary health care consumers. Coordination of care is one of the responsibilities of those in primary care. Physicians should exploit this role in making referrals to other providers and/or other programs that can offer needed services. These physicians can certainly incorporate many disease prevention/health promotion practices into their care, but there is no way a single physician can be adequately skilled and keep up with the services that will become increasingly available for promoting healthful behaviors (Nutting, 1986).

Referral is essential if preventive care is to be available at a reasonable cost. Referrals to other health providers and community support organizations can supply services more efficiently and at less cost (McGinnis et al., 1982), and it can be done equally well and more cheaply by health professionals with different training (Relman, 1982).

Dunn (1982) stated that other professionals such as nurses, health educators, and social workers are carrying out health promotion activities. He further concluded that extensive involvement of physicians in health promotion was not cost effective. McNamara (1982) reported that nurse practitioners and health educators can perform prevention related activities far more effectively than physicians.

McGinnis (1982) suggested one role of physicians was to refer patients to other health providers or community resources that can supply the necessary services more efficiently and/or at less cost. However, he added that traditional medical education does not prepare physicians to be comfortable making referrals, and their lack of familiarity with community resources contributes to this difficulty. McNamara (1982) supported the idea of referral, stating that many preventive services do not require the direct services of physicians and may be offered by those better trained and at less expense, such as nurse practitioners and/or health educators.

Campbell and Valente (1983, p. 284) suggested that physicians use "other health professionals" to provide reinforcement of the educational message. They identify other health professionals as office staff, nurses, or persons outside the office to whom the physician might refer. It is known that most individuals view physicians as the most credible source of health information, but is it realistic for them to be expected to provide all of the education and reinforcement necessary? They can be the ideal individuals to plant the seed (in a sense "prescribe") patient education.

Bartlett and Windsor (1985) predicted that an expanded relationship between health education and medicine could have the following positive outcomes: increased patient satisfaction with care, which would enhance the image of medicine in the community; improved patient compliance and decreased anxiety and fear, which may facilitate recovery; and reductions in malpractice suits as a result of better communication between provider and patient.

In summary, the need for health promotion/disease prevention activities in the primary care setting has been identified, the obstacles and barriers to incorporating health education into primary care settings are recognized, and a variety of efforts are being tried to overcome the many barriers in order to provide health promotion/disease prevention activities to the patients of primary care physicians. It has been suggested that health educators become an integral part of primary care referral practice. As reported by Grunberg & Hale (1988), a patient education service conducted by health educators for primary care physicians is feasible; and the time for it is long overdue.

REFERENCES

Altekruse, J. M. (1987). Viewpoint, President's message. *Perspectives on Prevention, 1*(2), 4–6.

American Medical Association Council on Scientific Affairs. (1983). Medical evaluations of healthy persons. *JAMA, 249,* 1626–1633.

Association of Teachers of Preventive Medicine. (1986, September). *Directory and Profile of Academic Units in Preventive Medicine.*

Barbour, D. J. (1987a). Outlook, Executive report. *Perspectives on Prevention, 1*(2), 7.

Barbour, D. J. (1987b). WASHINGTON, DC report on legislation and policy. *Perspectives on Prevention, 1*(2), 47.

Barker, W. H., & Jonas, S. (1981). The teaching of preventive medicine in American medical schools, 1940–1980. *Preventive Medicine, 10,* 674–688.

Bartlett, E. E. (1983). Reimbursement of patient education: More data . . . or more action? *Patient Education and Counseling, 5*(1), 4–5.

Bartlett, E. E. (1984). Health education in medical education. *Preventive Medicine, 14,* 100–114.

Bartlett, E. E., & Windsor, R. A. (1985). Health education and medicine: Competition or cooperation? *Health Education Quarterly, 12*(4), 219–229.

Beasley, J. W. (1987). Perspective of an academician in family medicine. *Perspectives on Prevention, 1*(2), 22–23.

Becker, M. H. (1985). Patient adherence to prescribed therapies. *Medical Care, 23*(5), 539–555.

Boynton, E. S. (1986, April). *Health risk behaviors among a medical faculty, a non-medical faculty and medical students.* Presentation: American Alliance for Health, Physical Education, and Dance. National Convention, city.

Brandt, E. N. *Toward a healthier america.* (1985). National Center for Health Promotion and Preventive Medicine. 660 West Redwood Street, Baltimore, MD. 21201

Brody, J. E. (1984). Taking charge of your health: The role of patients and professionals. *Patient Education in the Primary Care Setting Proceedings of the Seventh Annual Conference* (pp. 35–40). Kansas City: St. Mary's Hospital.

Center for Health Education, Inc. (CHE). (1983). The Brochure of the Center for Health Education, Inc. Baltimore, MD.

Calkins, D. R. (1987). Perspective of an academician in general internal medicine. *Perspectives on Prevention, 1*(2), 31–33.

Campbell, J. L., & Valente, C. M. (1983). Physician involvement in health education: needs, problems, solutions. *Maryland State Medical Journal, 32*(4), 284–290.

Clearie, A. F., Blair, S. N., & Ward, W. B. (1982, September). The role of the physician in health promotion: Findings from a community telephone survey. *The Journal of the South Carolina Medical Association,* 503–505.

Coffelt, C. F. (1987). Perspective of a OB/GYN practitioner. *Perspectives on Prevention, 1*(2), 36–37.

Cohn, V. (1985, November 6). Finding a health plan. *Washington Post Health,* pp. 14, 17.

David, A. K., & Boldt, J. S. (1980). A study of preventive health attitudes and behaviors in a family practice setting. *The Journal of Family Practice, 11,* 77–84.

DeMuth, N. M., Fielding, J. E., Stunkard, A. J., & Hollander, R. B. (1986). Evaluation of industrial health promotion programs: Return-on-investment and survival of the fittest. In M. F. Cataldo & T. J. Coates (Eds.), *Health and Industry: A Behavioral Medicine Perspective* (pp. 433–452). New York: John Wiley and Sons.

Dunn, M. R. (1982). Health promotion: The physician's role. *Public Health Reports, 97*(3), 229–232.

Faust, H. S. (1986). The HMO experience: Is clinical prevention feasible in the real world? *Perspectives on Prevention, 1*(1), 21–23.

Fleming, T. (1980). Wellness. *Postgraduate Medicine, 67*(2), 19, 21.

Fletcher, D. J. (1985). Building a pathway to better health: The primary care physician's role. *Postgraduate Medicine, 77*(1), 297–310.

Ford, A. S., & Ford, W. S. (1983). Health education and the primary care physician: the practitioner's perspective. *Social Science and Medicine, 17*(20), 1505–1512.

Fried, R. A. (1987). Prevention and primary care: The ice is melting. *Perspectives on Prevention, 1*(2), 8–9.

Glanz, K., Fiel, S. B., & Walber, L. R. (1982). Preventive health behavior of physicians. *Community, 57*(8), 637–639.

Green, K. (1985). Health promotion: Its terminology, concepts, and modes of practice. *Health Values: Achieving High Level Wellness, 9*(3), 8–14.

Green, L. W., Kreuter, M. W., Deeds, S. G., & Partridge, K. B. (1980). *Health Education Planning: A Diagnostic Approach.* Palo Alto, CA: Mayfield Publishing Company.

Greenberg, J. S., & Hale, J. F. (1988). The receptivity to and the feasibility of patient education for patients of private practice, primary care physician. *American Journal of Health Promotion 3*(2), 36–43.

Hankey, T. L. (1987). Perspective of a practitioner of family medicine. *Perspectives on Prevention, 1*(2), 24–26.

Harrell, J. UPDATE ODPHP. (1986). *Perspectives on Prevention, 1*(1), 31–32.

Harrell, J. UPDATE ODPHP. (1987). *Perspectives on Prevention, 1*(2), 45.

Haynes, R. B. (1979). Introduction. In R. B. Haynes, D. W. Taylor, & D. L. Sackett, (Eds.), *Compliance in Health Care* (pp. 11–19). Baltimore: Johns Hopkins University Press.

Inventory of knowledge and skills relating to disease prevention and health promotion. (1987). *Perspectives on Prevention, 1*(2), 14–18.

Isbister, C. (1976, January 24). Health services for women. *The Medical Journal of Australia, 1,* 94–95.

Jonas, S. (1981). Health oriented physician education. *Preventive Medicine, 10,* 700–709.

Kaplan, R. M. (1985). Behavioral epidemiology, health promotion, and health services. *Medical Care, 23*(5), 564–583.

Kehrer, B. H., Sloan, F. A., & Woolridge, J. (1984). Changes in primary medical care delivery, 1975–1979: Findings from the physician capacity utilization surveys. *Social Science and Medicine, 18*(98), 653–660.

Kernaghan, S. G., & Giloth, B. E. (1983). *Working With Physicians in Health Promotion: A Key to Successful Programs.* Chicago: American Hospital Association.

Kottke, T. E., Foels, J. K., Hill, C., Choi, T., & Fenderson, D. A. (1983). Perceived palatability of the prudent diet: Results of a dietary demonstration for physicians. *Preventive Medicine, 12,* 588–593.

La Vigne, P. (Ed.). (1980, April). Patient Education in the Primary Care Setting Proceedings of the Third Conference. Minneapolis: University of Minnesota.

Logsdon, D. N., Rosen, M. A., & Demak, M. M. (1982). The INSURE project on lifecycle preventive health services. *Public Health Reports, 97*(4), 308–317.

Logsdon, D. N., & Rosen, M. A. (1984). The cost of preventive health services in primary medical care and implications for health insurance coverage. *Journal of Ambulatory Care Management, 7*(4), 46–55.

Mendenhall, R. C. (1981). *Medical Practice in the United States.* Princeton, NJ: The Robert Wood Johnson Foundation.

McGinnis, J. M. (1980). Trends in disease prevention: assessing the benefits of prevention. *Bulletin New York Academy of Medicine, 56*(1), 38–44.

McGinnis, J. M., Moritsugu, K., & Roberts, C. M. (1982). Conference summary and discussion of future directions. *Public Health Reports, 97*(3), 241–243.

McNamara, D. G. (1982). Preventive health services: The physician's role. *Public Health Reports, 97*(3), 224–226.

McPhee, S. J. (1987). Perspective of a practitioner in general internal medicine. *Perspectives on Prevention, 1*(2), 34–35.

Mullen, K., & Costello, G. (1983), Primary care physicians as a source of health education needs assessment data. Unpublished report, Community Health Education Demonstration Project, Lexington County Hospital, West Columbia, SC.

Mullen, P. D., & Katayama, C. K. (1985). Health promotion in private practice: An analysis. *Family and Community Health, 8*(1), 79–87.

Murphy, L. R. (1984). Occupational stress management: a review and appraisal. *Journal of Occupational Psychology, 57,* 1–15.

Nutting, P. A. (1986). Health promotion in primary medical care: Problems and potential. *Preventive Medicine, 15,* 537–548.

O'Donnell, M. P., & Ainsworth, T. H. (Eds.). (1984). *Health Promotion in the Workplace.* New York: John Wiley & sons.

Orlandi, M. A. (1987). Promoting health and preventing disease in health care settings: An analysis of barriers. *Preventive Medicine, 16,* 119–130.

Orleans, C. T., George, L. K., Houpt, J. L., & Brodie, K. H. (1985). Health promotion in primary care: A survey of U.S. family practitioners. *Preventive Medicine, 14,* 636–647.

PASSING REVIEW reports on prevention from the field. (1986). *Perspectives on Prevention, 1*(1), 36–39.

PASSING REVIEW reports on prevention from the field. (1987a). *Perspectives on Prevention, 1*(2), 50–60.

PASSING REVIEW reports on prevention from the field. (1987b). *Perspectives on Prevention, 1*(3), 54–64.

Polakoff, P. L. (1982). Pathology vs. prevention: the health promotion debate. *Occupational Health and Safety, 51*(6), 13–15.

Prather, S. E. (1984). Making collaborative patient education work in a private obstetric/gynecology practice. *Patient Education in the Primary Care Setting: Proceedings of the Seventh Annual Conference, 7,* 65–70. Kansas City: St. Mary's Hospital.

Relman, A. S. (1982). Encouraging the practice of preventive medicine and health promotion. *Public Health Reports, 97*(3), 216–219.

Rentmeester, K. L. (1984). The economics of wellness promotion: Values versus economics. *Health Values: Achieving High Level Wellness, 8*(5), 6–9.

Rimer, B. K., Stretcher, V. J., Keintz, M., & Engstrom, P. F. (1986). A survey of physicians' views and practices on patient education for smoking cessation. *Preventive Medicine, 15,* 92–98.

Schneider, S. L. (1984). Organizing self-care programs that foster patient involvement. *Patient Education in the Primary Care Setting: Proceedings of the Seventh Annual Conference, 7,* 53–57. Kansas City: St. Mary's Hospital.

Scott, C. S., & Neighbor, W. E. (1985). Preventive care attitudes of medical students. *Social Science and Medicine, 21,* 299–305.

Simson, S., & Wilson, L. B. (1984). Education in prevention, health promotion and aging in medical and nursing schools. *Gerontology & Geriatrics Education, 3*(3), 43–52.

Sobal, J., Valente, C. M., Muncie, H. L., Levine, D. M., & Deforge, B. R. (1985). Physicians' beliefs about the importance of 25 health promoting behaviors. *American Journal of Public Health, 75*(12), 1427–1428.

Squyres, W. D. (1985). *Patient Education and Health Promotion in Medical Care.* Palo Alto: Mayfield Publishing.

U.S. Congress, House, Subcommittee on Health and the Environment of the Committee on Interstate and Foreign Commerce. (1976). *A Discursive Dictionary of Health Care.,* 94th Congress, 2nd session. Washington, DC: U.S. Government Printing Office.

U.S. Department of Health, Education, and Welfare. (1978, September). *Disease Prevention & Health Promotion: Federal Programs and Prospects. Report of the Departmental Task Force on Prevention* (DHEW [PHS] Publication No. 79-55071B). Washington, DC: U.S. Government Printing Office.

U.S. Department of Health, Education, and Welfare. (1979). *Healthy People: the Surgeon General's report on health promotion and disease prevention* (DHEW Publication No. 79-55071). Washington, DC: U.S. Government Printing Office.

U.S. Department of Health, Education, and Welfare. (1980a). *Living Well An Introduction to Health Promotion and Disease Prevention* (DHEW Publication No. 80-50121). Washington, DC: U.S. Government Printing Office.

U.S. Department of Health, Education, and Welfare. (1980b, April). *National Center for Health Statistics: The National Ambulatory Medical Care Survey, 1977 Summary* (Publication No. 80-1795). Washington, DC: U.S. Government Printing Office).

U.S. Department of Health and Human Services. (1984a). *Health Promotion and Disease Prevention in Primary Care.* Rockville, MD: National Center for Health Services Research.

U.S. Department of Health and Human Services. (1981). *Promoting Health/Preventing Disease: Objectives for the Nation.* Washington, DC: U.S. Government Printing Office.

U.S. Department of Health and Human Services. (1984b). *Proceedings of Prospects for a Healthier America: Achieving the Nation's Health Promotion Objectives.* Washington, DC: U.S. Government Printing Office.

U.S. Department of Health and Human Services. (1985). Provisional data from the health promotion and disease prevention supplement to the national health interview survey: United States, January–March 1985. *Advance Data from Vital and Health Statistics, 113,* 1–15. (DHHS Pub. No. [PHS] 86-1250). Hyattsville MD: Public Health Service.

Vartabedian, R. E., & Hamilton, T. E. (1982). Teaching preventive care in a family health center: How one residency does it. *Patient Education in the Primary Care Setting: Proceedings of the Fifth Annual Conference 5,* 79–81. Kansas City: St. Mary's Hospital.

Wechsler, H., Levin, S., & Idelson, R. K. (1983). The physician's role in health promotion: A survey of primary care practitioners. *New England Journal of Medicine, 308*(2), 97–100.

Weinberg, A., & Andrus, P. L. (1982). Continuing medical education: Does it address prevention? *Journal of Community Health, 7*(1), 211–214.

Wells, K. B., Lewis, C. E., Leake, B., Schleiter, M. K., & Brook, R. H. (1986). The practices of general and subspecialty internists in counseling about smoking and exercise. *American Journal of Public Health, 76,* 1009–1013.

Wolf, T. M., & Randall, H. M. (1987). A health promotion program for freshman medical students. In Network: Report on Departments of Preventive Medicine. *Perspectives on Prevention, 1*(3), 43.

Yoder, L. R., Jones, S. L., & Jones, P. K. (1985). The association between health care behavior and attitudes. *Health Values: Achieving High Level Wellness, 9*(4), 24–31.

INDEX